A–Z Dictionary of Wound Care

In association with Johnson & Johnson and Mark Allen Publishing Limited

Fiona Collins, Sylvie Hampton and Richard White

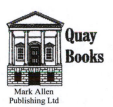

Quay Books

Mark Allen
Publishing Ltd

Quay Books Division, Mark Allen Publishing Limited,
Jesses Farm, Snow Hill, Dinton, Wiltshire, SP3 5HN

British Library Cataloguing-in-Publication Data
A catalogue record is available for this book

© Mark Allen Publishing Ltd 2002
ISBN 1 85642 225 9
First published 2002
First reprint 2003

Printed and bound in Great Britain by Biddles Ltd, *www.biddles.co.uk*

Contents

List of figures

About the authors

Sylvie Hampton was employed as Tissue Viability Nurse at Eastbourne for four years and Fiona Collins spent five years as a Senior Lecturer in Occupational Therapy at the University in Brighton. They formed a close relationship in research and clinical practice, which has naturally developed into a consultancy partnership in independent practice, Tissue Viability Consultancy Services Ltd (TVCS). TVCS has progressed with both practitioners developing their clinical skills by continuing to assess and treat patients and by consulting for nursing homes and the local Health Authority. They also regularly contribute articles to journals on the subjects of wound care and pressure ulcer prevention. A further aspect of their work includes assisting manufacturers of pressure reducing equipment and wound dressings in product development, preparation of marketing material and new product evaluation.

Richard White has thirty years' experience in dermatology and wound care having worked as a research scientist, university lecturer, and Associate Medical Director in the pharmaceutical industry. He has a number of publications related to skin biochemistry and physiology, dermatology, oral health and wound care. He now has his own company, Medical Communications, which provides medical writing, clinical research and medical marketing consultancy services.

TVCS and Medical Communications have developed a close alliance, enabling them to combine scientific, clinical and regulatory services for manufacturers, the NHS and private hospitals/nursing homes.

Acknowledgement

The authors wish to gratefully acknowledge the valuable contribution made by Dr Kate Springett in preparing this dictionary.

Foreword

How many times do we wonder the exact meaning of something that we have read or just heard? This can happen within any subject, and often the normal route for explanation would be the dictionary. So, why should wound care be any different?

Wound care is a vast topic that appears to be continually growing in complexity, with a plethora of new dressings and therapies and a demand for evidence-based practice. In order to evaluate the evidence when confronted with it, it is imperative to understand fully all of the terminology. What better way than through a specific wound care dictionary.

Unlike the traditional dictionary, this text expands beyond the direct definition of the word to give an understanding of its application to clinical practice; providing crucial information towards that all-important evidence-based practice. More importantly, the authors are a team of experts within the field of tissue viability and have the 'hands on' experience that allows them to appreciate the need for simple yet comprehensive explanations to this often complex field of practice.

I am sure that you will find this book an invaluable resource, providing accurate and accessible information both for reference and to complement daily practice.

Lorraine Jackson
Clinical Education Manager
Johnson & Johnson Wound Management

February 2002

Introduction

This dictionary has been designed to define words and terms that are used in tissue viability with the aim of providing clinical and evidence-based information in wound care and pressure ulcer prevention.

The dictionary definitions include words that are in common use in tissue viability and also those that are rarely used, but require explanation when discovered in academic journals. This reference book has been produced to assist nurses on tissue viability courses, students, physiotherapists, occupational therapists and those with a general interest in the subject. The definitions include the pure meaning of each word but also offer comment on the application within clinical practice. There are several pages of illustrations that support descriptions within the text and this will offer valuable assistance to the practitioner when undertaking wound assessments.

There are many biochemical terms within the text and these are intended to offer a better understanding of wound healing and provide background information for evidence-based practice (the art and science of wound care).

This first edition is intended as the foundation upon which successive revisions and updates will form a comprehensive wound care and tissue viability resource for all with an interest in the subject.

Fiona Collins
Sylvie Hampton
Richard White

November 2001

A

ABPI (SEE Ankle brachial pressure index).

Absorbent Substance which takes fluids up into its structure, or around its structure (adsorbent), eg. fluid will soak into cotton wool.

Acanthosis Changes in the stratum spinosum layer of the epidermis where it thickens. This is seen as a reaction to prolonged exposure to sunlight and can complicate or be complicated by chronic ulcer formation.

Acetate wound maps Clear sheets of acetate that are placed over the wound so that the outline of the wound can be traced and then used as a comparison for future mapping. It is a useful way to demonstrate healing in a wound. Difficulties are encountered when exudate contaminates the back of the sheet and when the wound moisture creates a mist on the sheet so that the wound outline cannot be identified. To prevent the sheet misting it can be wiped prior to application with an alcohol swab, which must be allowed to dry before application.

Actin A protein which unites with troponin and tropomyosin to form thin filaments in muscle.

Acute inflammatory oedema Oedema accompanied by the signs of infection with pain, redness, heat and swelling. Pitting will be absent because the fibrin network acts as a gel and traps the fluid. This can occur anywhere on the body and may give rise to ulceration.

Adenosine triphosphate (ATP) Within the cell, energy is released from glucose and stored in a high energy molecule — Adenosine triphosphate.

Adhesions Internal organs frequently adhere to each other. This leads to pain, occasional dysfunction and the need for repeat surgery. Localised scar tissue is a frequent outcome. This can occur for a number of reasons including surgery and infection. There is evidence that the use of hyaluronic films placed between the organs during surgery can avoid adhesions.

Adherence Inappropriately used wound dressings may adhere to a wound bed and cause trauma on removal.

Adipose tissue Food surplus to body requirements is laid down as fat stores (adipose tissue). It insulates the body against heat loss and protects and cushions internal organs. Adipose tissue can provide some protection of the bony prominences, and so help to prevent pressure ulcer development. The adipose layer is subcutaneous (below the dermal level).

Adrenocorticotrophic hormone (ACTH) A regulatory hormone, responsible for the release of glucocorticoids from the adrenal cortex.

Aerobic bacteria Some bacteria are dependent on oxygen for growth and these are called aerobic bacteria. The presence and colour of exudate within the wound may indicate the presence of aerobic bacteria. Some species such as *Pseudomonas* and *Staphylococci* also have a characteristic odour.

Aerobic organisms (SEE Aerobic bacteria).

Aetiology The cause and process of disease.

AgNO$_3$ Chemical formula for silver nitrate.

Alginate Alginate dressings are derived from algenic acid extracted from seaweed and create a hydrophilic gel in the presence of exudate. There is a high content of Ca^{2+} within alginate and this can be exchanged for sodium ions in the wound. When a blood vessel is damaged, a mixture of clotting factors utilises Ca^{2+} to initiate the clotting cascade; therefore, Ca^{2+} is an important part of stabilising a bleeding wound. Large numbers of reactions in the mitochondria are calcium-dependent and calcium can thus be regarded as an intracellular messenger by which particular reactions are speeded up while others are slowed. The transport of calcium across the mitochondria membrane is an important cellular control mechanism. All alginates have the capacity to act as a haemostat, although only one has been granted a license for use as such.

Allergen A substance that causes an immunological reaction, for example, by stimulating the biological activity of IgE which creates hypersensitivity reactions (hives, asthma, etc). Patients with leg ulcers are often exposed to high levels of allergens in the form of the many dressings that they are required to use. When an open wound is present (providing easy systemic access for any allergen), the leg ulcer patient has potential for hypersensitivity to dressings.

Aloe Vera Aloe Vera belongs to the lily family and its healing properties have been known for thousands of years The aloe plant is between 99 and 99.5% water with an average pH of 4.5 and 75 different ingredients including; vitamins, minerals, enzymes, sugars, sterols, amino acids and salicylic acid. There appears to be some value in using Aloe Vera and propolis in eczema, although this is anecdotal and unproven. Further information is required prior to using it for wound care.

Alogens Substances released following injury, associated with both pain and inflammation, including bradykinin, histamine and serotonin.

Alternating mattress A mattress with individual cells that inflate and deflate air. Cells inflate at different times with some mattresses providing alternately inflating and deflating cells and some with two inflated and one deflated cell. The inflation and deflation alternates in a cycle to ensure that interface pressure is relieved periodically. Mattress cycles vary from six minutes to ten minutes. The movement of the cells mimics movements of the patient, relieving pressure under the area of the deflated cell. This type of mattress is indicated in very high risk patients and those with established pressure ulcers. Proactive use of effective pressure redistributing (SEE Pressure reducing) mattresses, ie. static mattresses will lead to a more cost-effective selection of dynamic air mattresses.

Amorphous (SEE Hydrogel).

Anaemia A deficiency of red blood cells or a reduction in the quality of the red blood cells. The haemoglobin red pigment in red blood cells is used for carrying oxygen. (SEE Haemoglobin.) Diagnosis is confirmed when haemoglobin levels fall below 13 grams per 100 millilitres in males and below 12 grams in non-pregnant women. This leads to a lowered potential for transporting oxygen to the tissues. The result of this is a reduction in the energy available for wound repair, thereby delaying or preventing wound healing. Immunity may also be compromised, as leucocytes, macrophages, etc require oxygen to function. If the defence cells are not functioning the bacteria will be able to proliferate, increasing the potential for clinical infection. (SEE Sickle cell anaemia.)

Anaerobic Without oxygen.

Anaerobic bacteria Bacteria that thrive in an oxygen free environment. These micro-organisms bury under necrotic tissue and provide some of the pungent malodour in these wounds. The malodour is due to the volatile fatty acids that are the products of bacterial metabolism. Examples are *Bacteroides spp.* and *Chlostridia*. (SEE Malodour.)

Anaerobic organisms (SEE Anaerobic bacteria).

Analgesic A substance given systemically or topically, that relieves pain. Topical anaesthetic creams are not yet licensed for wound care. (SEE Topical anaesthesia.)

Anaphylaxis An immunological reaction, immediate hypersensitivity. A rapid over-exaggerated response to a systemic or topical allergen which can result in total suppression of respiration or cardio-vascular function. Mild anaphylactic reactions manifest as localised urticaria and pruritus.

Anastomosis A surgical joining of two branches of a blood vessel or connection of two hollow structures, eg. gut.

Angiogenesis The production of new blood vessels. In a wound new vessels grow into a loop and when seen in the lighter pink connective tissue of the wound bed, they have the appearance of deep red granules — this is called granulation tissue and is a feature of a healing wound.

Angiogram A radiological examination of arteries using a contrast medium. This examination can identify atherosclerosis in patients with leg ulcers and can lead to angioplasty or femoral popliteal by-pass.

Angioplasty A surgical method of removing atherosclerosis from the lumen of arteries. When successful, this can have a rapid effect on the healing of arterial ulcers.

Ankle brachial pressure index (ABPI) Ankle brachial pressure index is a calculation of arterial efficiency using Doppler ultrasound (*Figure 1*). The measure-ment is achieved by using the highest systolic pressure recorded in the ankle and dividing it by the highest systolic pressure in the arm. (Place A (ankle) over B (brachial) $130/120 \cong 1.0$ or ABPI >1). The result in normal arterial flow should be ABPI 1.0. and this would be a safe level to use compression therapy. However, some patients will have mixed aetiology of venous and arterial disease and may still be safe for compression. The lowest 'safe' level for compression is thought to be >0.8. Lower than 0.8 is unsafe for compression. (SEE Critical limb ischaemia.)

Ankle flare A tiny dilation of superficial blood vessels on the medial aspect of the foot, is often a precursor to venous ulceration.

Anoxia Absence of oxygen from arterial blood tissues or organs. Different from hypoxia (SEE Hypoxia.)

Anterior Facing the front of the body.

Anterior pelvic tilt A normal forward movement of the pelvis in the antero-posterior plane. In functional sitting, the anterior tilt is adopted when a person sits forwards. In some instances a person may develop a tendency to adopt this sitting position as opposed to the normal sitting position (SEE Normal sitting), due to causes such as flexion contractures at the hip joint, hypertonicity of the hip flexors and weak abdominal muscles. Anterior pelvic tilt is frequently seen in people with muscular dystrophy or spina bifida. This position can result in postural changes: the pelvis rocks forwards, and the ischial tuberosities push backwards, potentially placing weight onto the pubis increasing risk of pressure sore development. As the pelvis moves forwards, the hip angle closes, increasing the risk of flexion contractures of the hip. The femurs medially rotate and adduct. The spine and trunk are forced forwards, increasing lumbar lordosis and the shoulder girdle becomes retracted.

Anterior superior iliac spines (ASISs) These are located on the anterolateral aspect of the pelvis, below the iliac crests. They can be located by either palpating anteriorly and inferiorly from the iliac crests, or by palpating the area where the pelvis and thighs meet. The ASISs are slightly hooked, and this approach allows the assessor to locate them. In a neutral sitting position, the ASISs are level with each other when palpated from an anterior position, indicating that weight is being taken evenly on both ischial tuberosities.

Anterior tibial artery An artery that runs down over the mid-dorsum of the foot. (SEE Dorsalis pedis.)

Antibacterial A substance with bactericidal or bacteristatic properties. 'Kills' or 'inhibits' bacteria, eg. an antiseptic.

Antibiotic A chemical substance, produced by a micro-organism which has the capacity, in dilute solutions, to inhibit selectively the growth of, or to kill, other micro-organisms. Sir Alexander Fleming discovered penicillin in mould in 1928 and led the way to production of antibiotic drugs and the belief that these may eradicate infectious disease by destroying bacteria. However, bacteria are an example of Darwin's theory of 'survival of the fittest'. In 1961, following over-enthusiastic administration of antibiotics world-wide, methicillin-resistant *Staphylococcus aureus* (MRSA) was reported for the first time as indiscriminate use of antibiotics led to the selection of new resistant strains of bacteria. Topical antibiotics are no longer advised due to the potential for resistant strains to occur. Systemic antibiotics should only be given when clinical infection has been identified.

Anticoagulant Prevents blood from clotting. (SEE Heparin and Warfarin.)

Antiembolism stockings Stockings (hosiery) that provide moderate compression (Class I–II) and assist venous return in immobile patients. These reduce the risk of deep vein thrombosis and pulmonary embolism. These stockings are recommended for all those considered at risk and who are undertaking long-haul air travel. Caution should be taken using this type of hosiery when arterial disease is suspected.

Antigens Small molecules of a 'non-self' substance, ingested or topical, which attach to cell-surface (membrane) receptor sites. If they attach to cells involved in the inflammatory response, then clinical features of inflammatory reaction will develop. This can sometimes be seen around a wound site, with erythema that outlines the shape of the dressing.

Antimicrobial This is a vague non-specific term used to describe a substance that destroys microbes, or prevents their growth and multiplication. (SEE Antibacterial.)

Antiseptic A substance used for sterilising or reducing the growth of bacteria. Antiseptics commonly used in wound care are iodine and chlorhexidine.

Apoptosis Self-destruction of cells. A distinctive death of cells that could more accurately be described as cell suicide. Programmed cell death, part of the normal process of control of growth.

Apposition Bringing together two structures, ie. through wound suture.

Approximation A wound that has the edges brought together in approximation will heal through primary intention. (SEE Primary intention.)

Aqueous Pertains to water, for example, aqueous cream, a cream used to cleanse and maintain skin integrity.

Arachis oil Peanut oil used to soften hyperkeratosis. Great care should be taken when applying this oil as there is a risk that the patient may be allergic to nuts.

Armrests The height of the armrests in an armchair or wheelchair should be high enough for the elbows to be comfortably supported with the shoulders in a neutral position. If they are too high, the shoulders will be hunched and there is a potential to develop pressure ulcers on the elbows; if too low, the shoulders will be depressed, and inadequate support will be provided for the arms, resulting in reduced sitting stability. The armrest should be covered in a soft material, eg. foam to provide comfort.

Arnica Homeopathic preparation, often in cream form, used to soothe soft tissue discomfort and reduce bruising. It should not be applied to a wound.

Art and science of nursing The art of nursing is formed through experience, reflective practice and skill. The science of nursing is based on research evidence, and requires knowledge, understanding, and an enquiring mind.

Arterial insufficiency The lumen of the artery becomes smaller due to athero-sclerosis and arteriosclerosis, with less blood being delivered to the lower extremities.

Arterial perfusion The movement of blood through tissues or organ via the blood vessels. Poor perfusion of the feet could indicate arterial disease and pre-dispose to ulceration in the leg and feet.

Arterial ulcers Ulcers that are formed anywhere on the leg or feet, due to arterial insufficiency. These wounds are often related to pain, particularly at night, and have a 'stamped out' appearance. Patients frequently report pain relief with the limbs in a dependent position. Arterial ulcers will often be symmetrical in shape and have steep, caved sides.

Asepsis Without pathogens, infections or toxins. Aseptic technique is designed to prevent bacteria from reaching vulnerable sites through use of sterile techniques. The method of achieving asepsis relies on excellent hand washing techniques, use of sterile equipment and a non-touch technique when caring for acute wounds or cathe-terisation. The use of forceps for cleansing wounds in aseptic procedures is no longer recommended as the hardness of the forceps can damage newly forming tissue. Asepsis is unnecessary with chronic wounds, which are invariably colonised.

ASIS (SEE Anterior superior iliac spine).

Assessment Information obtained via observation, questioning, physical examin-ation and clinical investigations in order to establish a baseline for planning intervention.

Atherosclerotic arteries Fatty de-generative plaques of fat are deposited on the walls of arteries and harden. The layers of plaque are laid down until the walls of the arteries are no longer elastic. Atherosclerosis can be heard with a Doppler ultrasound as there will be no 'rebound' sounds and the only sound to be heard is a distinctive monophasic 'woof-woof' sound as if a dog is barking. Due to

the hardened walls the artery may not be compressible with a sphygmomanometer pressure cuff, and this can give false elevated ankle pressure readings. Any ankle reading that is wildly elevated, with a monophasic sound should be suspected of arterial disease. Referral to a vascular consultant would be advisable in such circumstances.

Atherosclerosis Fatty deposits. (SEE Atherosclerotic arteries.)

ATP (SEE Adenosine triphosphate).

Atrophie blanche Small (1–3 cm diameter) avascular areas of scarring on the skin often associated with a history of ulceration. Can be found near established ulcers or in areas of haemosiderin and in the gaiter area. The physical appearance is a white or grey area of tissue. The pathological process seems to involve thrombosis and the obliteration of capillaries in the middle and deep dermis.

Audit Audit investigates present clinical practice and asks the question, 'is this best clinical practice?' It is an important method of monitoring and implementing change. For example, prevalence or incidence can be audited and used as an indication of improve-ments in standards of care.

Auto-immune diseases Immunological disorders where the body's immune system attacks the tissues, recognising them as 'foreign'. An example is rheumatoid arthritis which can result in vasculitis and ulceration (*Figure 2*). Multiple sclerosis is also an autoimmune disease which carries a high risk of pressure ulcers, due to:

- ❖ immobility
- ❖ physiological vascular impairment
- ❖ poor seated posture.

Autologous (autograft) One's own self, eg. for an autologous skin graft, skin is taken from another site on the same person.

Autolysis Is the body's own natural capacity for removing necrotic tissue as it uses its own enzymes to lyse, or break-down, devitalised tissue. In wound care autolysis is encouraged through the use of 'moist wound' dressings, such as hydrocolloids, or hydrogels.

Autonomic neuropathy A degenerative disorder of the autoimmune nervous system which leads to loss of blood flow to the feet

and loss of the sweating response, often associated with diabetes. Can lead to diabetic foot ulceration.

Avascular No (or few) blood vessels are present in the tissue.

B

Backrest When sitting each person will require a different backrest height, according to his medical and functional needs. A higher backrest is more supportive and should be used for the elderly, and those with poor trunk and head control as this increases sitting stability, decreasing the risk of poor seated posture which results in pressure ulcer development.

Back-slab Plastic or plaster splint that is used to support limbs, inhibit motion and reduce joint range of motion. A useful tool in the treatment of some diabetic ulcers as the plaster can be designed to relieve pressure in selected areas and removed for dressing change. The plaster is also fitted to the shape of the foot and this redistributes pressure away from pressure points.

Bacteraemia Bacteria that enters the blood stream. Identified through blood cultures. Can make the patient unwell. (SEE Septicaemia.)

Bactericidal Kills bacteria.

Bacteriostatic Prevents bacteria from reproducing and therefore allows the body's natural defences to reduce bacterial numbers, removing the potential for clinical infection.

Barrier function The stratum corneum layer of the skin is the primary barrier against the environment. Wound dressings and ointments may also incorporate a material to provide this protective function.

Basal cell carcinoma Also known as a rodent ulcer. A tumour that invades local

tissues, often with the appearance of a wart. Frequently presents as an ulcer that fails to heal. Rarely metastatic. Note that basal cell carcinoma can be a differential diagnosis in chronic ulceration.

Basement membrane (SEE Dermo-epidermal junction).

Bedsore Old-fashioned name for pressure ulcers. Pressure damage was always associated with long-term bed rest and therefore, these ulcers were called bedsores. There is a better understanding of cause and effect today, and it is known that a large percentage of pressure ulcers occur when patients are seated and so the use of the term 'bedsore' has been abandoned (*Figure 3*).

Beta-haemolytic *streptococci*
Bacteria which invade tissues readily, form a watery, serous exudate, and wounds infected with beta-haemolytic *streptococcus* often have eroded margins. (SEE Necrotising fasciitis.)

Bexhill armrests A wheelchair accessory designed to provide support to a hemiplegic arm and shoulder joint. Its use will reduce shoulder pain on the affected side without restricting mobility, and decrease the occurrence of tissue damage caused by a flacid arm being caught in a wheel of a wheelchair.

Bifurcation Site where, for example, blood vessels divide into two.

Bilateral Both (opposite) sides. For instance, ulcers on both legs would be bilateral ulcers.

Bioburden The amount of bacteria within a wound. The number of bacteria in a wound has an influence on potential of clinical infection — generally, the greater the number ($>10^5$) the greater the potential for infection to occur. (SEE Quorum sensing.)

Bio-engineered tissue Animal (probably human) tissue that is grown in a laboratory using cultured cells. For example, fibroblast dermal replacement and keratinocyte epidermal replacement.

Biofilm A membrane of glycocalyx that is secreted by highly organised bacterial communities. Biofilms may favour organism survival and decrease the effectiveness of topical and systemic antibacterial therapy.

Biopsy Small piece of tissue that is removed from any part of the body for diagnostic purposes.

Biosurgery Removal of slough or debridement of necrotic tissue or slough through larvae (maggot) therapy (*Figure 4*). (SEE Larval therapy.)

Bi-phasic sound Two distinct sounds of arterial blood flow heard through Doppler ultrasound assessment. In a young, healthy person, there would be three distinct sounds (tri-phasic) as the arteries are expanded by the rush of blood and then recoil and rebound. As the artery ages and wall elasticity reduces, there is often only the two (or bi-phasic) sounds. As atherosclerosis occurs, the sound may reduce to one. (SEE Monophasic.)

Black wound The stage of healing or non-healing is sometimes identified through wound colour. This is a subjective method and is not accurate but can be helpful in noting wound changes during assessment and documentation. A black wound (*Figure 5*) is generally a necrotic wound and requires debridement before the healing process will commence. (SEE Red wound, Yellow wound, Green wound, Pink wound.)

Blanching Skin whitens under compression due to local occlusion or vasoconstriction of the blood supply.

Blanching hyperaemia An area of erythema that turns white under finger pressure (SEE Erythema). When a bony prominence compresses the skin tissues against a hard surface (ie. the ischial tuberosities when in a seated position) the local blood supply will almost certainly be occluded and this leads to a blanching of the tissues. When the pressure is removed from the area the capillaries over-react and flush bright red. This is known as reactive hyperaemia and is a healthy counteraction to the original occlusion. At this point, there is no lasting damage to the capillaries or to local tissues. Blanching hyperaemia could be used as a warning sign of patient risk. If the blanching redness does not fade within a few minutes, then it is important to consider a higher-grade mattress for this patient. When ignored, blanching hyperaemia can progress to tissue damage. Blanching hyperaemia is difficult to detect in dark or tanned skin. (SEE Non-blanching hyperaemia.)

Blind randomised control trial A randomised study that does not permit the researcher to know which product is being applied or analysed. Relies on the ability of the study to provide two different items that appear identical when used. The researcher uses numbers to identify which product is used. This is simply achieved in drug trials by using a placebo that appears identical to the trial drug. It is a difficult criteria to achieve when dressings or mattresses are used as few are identical. (SEE RCTs.)

Blisters The result of a separation of the dermal and epidermal layers when the space between the two layers fills with fluid. Generally occur following friction, shear or disease. (SEE Burn blister.)

Bony prominence Projections of bone such as ischial tuberosities, greater trochanter, calcaneum and humerus, etc. As a result of this, tissue over bony prominences is frequently thin, increasing the risk of damage due to pressure sores.

Botulism After absorption into the bloodstream, botulinum toxin binds irreversibly to the presynaptic nerve endings, where it inhibits the release of acetylcholine. Diplopia, blurred vision, dysarthria, dysphagia, respiratory failure and paresis of the limbs are common symptoms of this intoxication. Botulism has been found in some honey so if honey is to be used in wound care, it is necessary to apply one that has been licensed for open wounds.

Braden risk assessment A method of assessing patient risk in the prevention of pressure ulcers. The assessment has given parameters and the results, when totalled, give a risk score (SEE *Appendix*).

Bradykinins These are vasoactive chemicals which are part of the inflammation and healing process. They are derived from plasma and contribute to prolonged vascular permeability. They are also chemical mediators that are important in the synthesis of granulation tissue.

Bullae sing. bulla. Another term for blisters.

Burn blister Burn blisters generally occur when heat separates the epidermis from the dermis. Fluid collects in the space that is left between the two levels and a blister is formed. De-roofing blisters may be harmful and can open the wound to clinical infection. The fluid can be withdrawn using a fine needle. However, larger blisters, involving necrotic tissue, must be debrided, particularly in the case of burns. Patients with large burns, requiring hospitalisation, are likely to be admitted to specialist units with expertise in caring for extensive burns.

C

Cachexia In a very poor state of health.

Cadexomer pastes Are compounds which slowly release free iodine from the powder base (carbohydrate) and doses the wound in iodine over a prolonged 72-hour period.

Calamine Topically applied preparation containing zinc. Used to soothe itchy and inflamed skin. Is available as a lotion or ointment.

Calcification It is possible for small patches of bone-like calcification to grow within a chronic and long-standing wound (*Figure 6*). These patches of bone require removal to allow granulation and epithelialisation to occur.

Calcinosis Deposition of calcium salts in various tissues of the body (seen in systemic sclerosis, rheumatoid arthritis). Can lead to tissue breakdown and ulceration.

Calciphylaxis A rare disorder of small-vessel calcification and cutaneous infarction associated with chronic renal failure. Also reported in conjunction with breast cancer, alcoholic cirrhosis and hyperparathyroidism. The lesion can appear as a chronic ulcer which becomes necrotic and fulminates. The pathophysiology has been attributed to protein C deficiency and thrombosis.

Calcium Large numbers of reactions in the mitochondria are calcium-dependent, and calcium can be regarded as an intracellular messenger by which particular reactions are speeded up while others are slowed down. The transport of calcium across the mitochondrial membrane can be seen as an important cellular control mechanism. Calcium, cation (Ca^{2+}), is intimately involved in the clotting cascade and is involved in haemostasis.

Calcium alginates (SEE Alginates).

Calendula Topically applied herbal preparation, derived from marigolds. It is used to soothe itchy and inflamed skin and to encourage healing. Insufficient information is currently available about its effect on wounds.

Calf venous pump Veins are unable to independently facilitate blood return to the heart and normal venous return requires the calf muscle to compress the deep veins during exercise. This action, known as the calf muscle pump or calf venous pump, increases pressure in the deep veins by 'squeezing', and in the superficial veins through vacuum action from the deeper system. As the calf muscle relaxes the pressure ceases and blood is prevented from returning to the lower extremities by the venous valves. A similar action is created by the pressure of the foot against the ground during walking. These mechanisms are the most important way of returning blood to the heart. Loss of ankle flexion, muscle wastage and immobility in the elderly reduces calf pump efficiency and predisposes to ulceration.

Calliper (Harpenden) A tool for measuring the thickness of the skin. May be useful in establishing a risk parameter for pressure ulcer prevention. Regularly used in dermatology for assessing skinfold thickness.

Callus Hard skin (alternative terms; callosity, callous, hyperkeratosis), can predispose to ulceration in the foot. When present, this tissue should be debrided by a professional with the appropriate education, qualifications and experience.

Calor Latin term for 'heat' as perceived in inflammation.

Candida albicans A yeast-like fungi that can cause an infection; sometimes known as thrush. Occurs in warm, moist areas of the body (under breasts, vagina, groin and mouth) and can be painful. One causative factor can be administration of systemic antibiotics, immunosuppressives and disease states, such as AIDS. Treatable with anti-fungal cream.

Candidiasis Infection by the yeast candida, often occurs in moist body flexures.

Capillary A capillary is a minute blood vessel that is the link between the arterial system and the venous system, creating a capillary network. Capillary walls are composed of selectively permeable endothelial cells. It is at the level of the capillary that haemostasis occurs and nutrients and oxygen are supplied to the tissues. It is also the capillaries that provide the 'loops' known as granulation tissue in a healing wound.

Carbamazepine A drug that is used to treat epilepsy but can also reduce pain. This makes it useful in painful wounds as it does not cause sleepiness.

Carbon dressings Carbon dressings contain activated charcoal which has the ability to absorb odour. Carbon can be found in certain foam dressings and plain dressings. One carbon dressing contains silver ions. This dressing not only reduces odour in a wound but also destroys bacteria through the use of silver. It can be used as a primary dressing although it is often used mistakenly as a secondary dressing, with the aim of eliminating odour.

Cell migration Cells that independently mobilise across a space. An example is epithelial tissue which migrates over granulation tissue in the final stages of healing. (SEE Epithelial tissues.)

Cell mitosis The division of cells.

Cellulitis Inflammation and infection of the cells, associated with redness, heat, swelling and pain. It can arise from minute, pinprick wounds, where the primary source of infection is difficult to find, such as a break in the skin between the toes. It is caused by various bacteria but group A *Streptoccoci* and *Staphylococcus aureus* are the most common agents (*Figure 7*).

Centre of gravity Pertaining to seating, the centre of gravity should be maintained in front of the spine in order to maximise sitting stability.

Cephalosporins Broad spectrum antibiotics (eg. Cefalexin) which target the cell wall of Gram-positive bacteria and interfere with the cell's osmotic pressure. This ensures that the cells cannot function, collapse occurs and the cell dies. Used in the treatment of septicaemia.

Charcoal dressing (SEE Carbon dressings).

Charcot joint Very common in diabetes. The main characteristic of the Charcot joint is a flattening of the medial longitudinal arch, often with a 'rocker bottom' shape to the foot. Build up of callosities causes abnormal pressure loading on the tissues and can often lead to ulceration. A wound over a Charcot joint can be very difficult to treat as it is, necessarily, a weight-bearing joint and osteoporosis, hyperostosis, osteolysis, pathological fracture, spontaneous dislocation of the joint and generalised joint or bone damage can occur. A well designed backslab fibreglass boot, or total contact cast can be an excellent way of relieving pressure during mobilisation.

Charing Cross four-layer system
Multi-layer (or four- or five-layer) bandaging developed as a result of research within Charing Cross Hospital, where use of multilayered bandaging suggested that a high rate of ulcer healing could be achieved in 12 weeks. The system of bandages contain orthopaedic wool, a crepe bandage, a long-stretch bandage and a cohesive bandage. Currently, there is no evidence to differentiate healing rates achieved with this system and a short-stretch compression system.

Chemical debridement Chemicals, such as hypochlorites and hydrogen peroxide, were once commonly used for chemical debridement. These have now been shown to be painful, become absorbed by the tissues and can cause disruption to some metabolic systems. They can be damaging to healing tissue and are not as effective as modern wound dressings. Chemicals are not recommended for debridement.

Chemical mediator A mediator is a molecule that is summoned during an inflammatory response and has a direct role to effect that response.

Chemokines A class of pro-inflammatory cytokines that has the ability to attract and activate leucocytes. Presence of these substances encourage cells into increased activity.

Chemokinesis A response by a motile cell to a soluble chemical that results in movement. These functions are important in the early stages of wound healing.

Chemotactic factors Substances produced as part of the inflammatory reaction which attract various cells (eg. macrophages) to the site of injury.

Chemotaxis In inflammation, the movement of cells to the site of injury in response to the release of chemotactic factors.

Chemotherapy The use of chemicals, and drugs such as antibiotics to treat disease. The term chemotherapy is sometimes mis-used as an exclusive treatment for cancer. Chemotherapy for cancer is with cytotoxic drugs which often have a specific action.

Chlorhexidine Antiseptic in common use for skin wash, mouth wash and in anti-bacterial dressings, not always effective against Methicillin-resistant *Staphylococcus aureus*. There are concerns about increasing resistance and in the overall use of antiseptic solutions.

Chronic wound A wound that has remained unhealed for more than six weeks. The reasons for delayed healing are complex and multiple with many overlapping factors such as underlying pathology, malnutrition, pressure, etc.

Cigarette smoking (SEE Smoking).

Clinical Governance A method of setting standards, monitoring and disseminating good practice. The aim is to ensure that clinical excellence is uniform and that all those responsible for health care follow guidelines of good practice. (SEE NICE.)

Clinical infection The presence of multiplying bacteria within the local tissues (SEE Infection). Generally has signs and symptoms of pyrexia, cellulitis, increasing malodour, pain and the patient has malaise. Clinically infected wounds should always be treated systemically. Choice of dressing is almost irrelevant until cellulitis is under control with antibiotics. Infected wounds have delayed healing even with the most advanced dressings. The selected dressing should rapidly remove bacteria from the surface of the wound. Clinical infection cannot be accurately detected through swabs as the results are taken from wound exudate, which is nearly always contaminated, and may not reflect the bacteria contained within the local tissues. Accurate results can be obtained through biopsy, but this is generally considered unwise.

Clotting cascade Complex sequence of chemical interactions which have the end result that fibrin is created to form a clot following vessel injury.

Cohesive bandage Bandages that have the ability to cling to themselves and do not require adhesive tape. Frequently used as the outermost layer of the four-layer bandaging system.

Collagen This is the most abundant protein in the animal world and is responsible for holding the body together, skeleton included. The term collagen is frequently used to mean collagen fibres, but actually relates to a family of glyco-proteins found in a range of histological entities, including collagen fibres, reticulin fibres, and basement membranes and may be detected in a wound within the first ten hours post-injury. Collagen is laid down and modified during the proliferative and maturation phases of wound healing.

Collagen matrix In the mature dermis cross-linked collagen forms a complex matrix which acts as a scaffold for fibroblasts, blood vessels and nerves.

Collagenase Proteolytic enzyme which breaks down native collagen as opposed to generic. Collagenases from mammalian cells are metalloenzymes and are collagen-type specific. Collagenases are involved in tissue breakdown and remodelling in wound healing.

Colonisation Multiplication of organisms in a wound without host reaction.

Commensal Bacteria which resides on or within a host without causing a reaction from the host.

Compatibility Drugs or topical substances which can be used together with no ill effects.

Compliance A measure of whether a patient follows treatment as prescribed.

Compression Compression therapy is becoming known as the main treatment option for venous ulceration, as research and experience has demonstrated the effectiveness of short-stretch, multi-layer (four- or five-layer) and long-stretch bandages. These methods of bandaging increase venous return, allowing the lower extremity tissues to recover from the effects of venous hypertension and offer a faster healing rate. Other methods of compression are UNNA boot (used mainly in America) and intermittent compression therapy (a boot operated by a compressor that is worn for an hour three times daily).

Compression hosiery This is supplied in three strengths (classes) in the UK. Class I is light compression (10mmHg–14mmHg). Class II is slightly higher compression (15mmHg–23mmHg) and is for prevention of venous ulceration. Class III is high compression (24mmHg–39mmHg) and can be used for treatment of venous ulcer-ation. Class II and III (the latter in particular) require Doppler ultrasound assessment prior to application of the stocking. In Europe, higher class stockings (IV and V) are used.

Compression stockings (SEE Compression hosiery).

Cone of pressure Pressure ulcers occur when pressure between a firm surface and a bony prominence compresses the tissues between and occludes the blood supply. The pressure is always greater nearer the bone where the initial damage occurs. The lesser pressure near the surface will gradually become apparent. Pressure damage is not seen until three or eight days after the initial damage occurs.

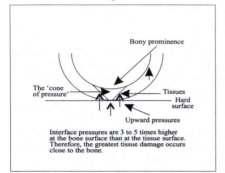

Interface pressures are 3 to 5 times higher at the bone surface than at the tissue surface. Therefore, the greatest tissue damage occurs close to the bone.

Connective tissue A general term for tissue derived from mesoderm. May be specialised as in bone and cartilage. Rich in extracellular matrix components, connective tissue surrounds or supports more highly ordered tissues and organs. The dermis is an example; this supports the epidermis and contains blood vessels and nerves. It has a high tensile strength provided by collagen. There are more than 14 genetically distinct collagens, encoded by 30 different genes which account for 70–80% of the dry weight of the dermis.

Contact dermatitis A dermatitis occurs when a patient becomes sensitive to something that touches the skin — dressings, topically applied substances, jewellery, soap, etc. Occasionally, patients appear to become sensitive to their own exudate and any dressing that holds the exudate against the peri-wound area will increase potential for a sensitivity reaction. With non-healing leg ulcers, in particular, contact dermatitis (sub-clinical or overt) may be a causative factor.

Contamination Organisms present within wound exudate but not multiplying or clinically affecting the host.

Contraction Contraction is a key stage in wound healing. Prior to contraction, the wound may appear to enlarge as it enters a healing phase. Granulation tissue is then laid down and grows toward the surface of the wound. As this is progressing, the wound edges will begin to contract in toward the centre. This is enhanced through the growth of epithelial tissue that begins to advance over the newly formed granulation tissue. It is thought that myofibroblasts present in this granulation tissue are responsible for contraction.

Contractures A fixation of the joint, often permanent, caused by a reduction in length of muscle fibres. Often associated with burns.

Corn (SEE Callus).

Corticosteroids A group of drugs used frequently in autoimmune disorders for their anti-inflammatory properties. They have a number of side-effects, including impeding the immune response and causing the skin and deeper tissues to be less tough and resilient than normal. They cause atrophy of the epidermis and superficial dermis and are thought to impair the later stages of wound healing.

Creams Used as a base vehicle for topical active ingredients, or alone as an emollient. They provide an oily layer over the surface of the skin which traps water underneath it, so 'moisturising' the skin. Creams contain water: this can support microbial growth therefore preservatives are required. These can cause allergic reactions.

Crepe bandage An extensible bandage that is used to support dressings or as one layer of a multi-layer bandage system. Cannot be used for compression in its own right as it loses 40% to 60% tension within 20 minutes.

Crepitus A sensation of crackling on tissue and joint palpation, may be felt in marked infection.

Criteria The basis on which to form decisions or a standard to be achieved. Points or parameters to consider, measure, etc.

Critical colonisation A term applied to the situation where host defences fail to maintain the balance of organisms in a wound at colonisation.

Critical limb ischaemia A point at which viability within the limb is at acute risk due to insufficiency of blood delivery, ie. when the limb becomes non-viable through insufficient blood flow, the ABPI may be 0.5 or less. When this occurs the limb will blanch when raised; upon lowering, the limb blanching persists (Buerger's sign).

Cultured dermis (SEE Bio-engineered tissue).

Cushions Cushions may be used in armchairs or wheelchairs. They are either for pressure-reducing or pressure-relieving purposes. When used in conjunction with armchairs they should be integral to the seat rather than as an addition. (SEE Pressure reducing; Pressure relieving.)

Cushioning In tissue viability cushioning would be associated with prevention of pressure in shoes, seating or mattresses through the use of foam and other materials.

Cyanosis This is a visible sign of cardiovascular disease and is usually accompanied by poor mobility. Poor oxygenation of the blood, distinguished by a blue tinge to the skin, nail beds and mucous membranes. It indicates a lack of available oxygen in the tissues. The presence of cyanosis has implications for wound healing as cell repair requires oxygen. (SEE Hypoxia.)

Cytokines Cytokines are small biological factors, such as some growth factors, that are delivered to the wound during episodes of inflammation. Cytokines are summoned to the wound by various components of inflammation, such as macrophages, platelets, etc. They are key mediators of the inflammatory phase, immune response, cell-cell interaction and communication. The term tends to be used for lymphokines, interferons, interleukins and TNF. (SEE Growth factors.)

Cytotoxic drugs Cytotoxic drugs destroy newly forming cells and this is of value in reducing mutant rapid growth tumours. However, there is a potential for these drugs also to destroy newly forming non-mutant cells, such as those required in wound healing. Therefore, healing will be delayed.

D

Debridement Taken from the French *débridement*, or *débrider* to remove adhesions. Literally: the surgical removal of devitalised, or contaminated tissue. Can be sharp (scalpel, scissors), chemical, or enzymatic debridement, larval therapy (maggots) or debridement through autolysis.

Decubitus ulcer (SEE Pressure ulcer).

Deep dermal burns (SEE Deep-partial thickness burn).

Deep tension sutures Deep tension sutures take a large 'bite' of tissue to relieve pressure on the normal suture line. Used when a wound is threatening to dehisce. This sometimes occurs, for example, in obese patients.

Deep vein thrombosis Deep vein thrombosis (DVT) occurs mainly in the deep veins within the calf muscle. Blood stasis, viscous blood and valvular dysfunction are the three predisposing factors (Virchow's triad). Blood stasis occurs when standing or sitting for long periods. Viscous blood occurs within smokers, those taking oral contraception, during air travel due to dehydration and in those who are unwell. Valvular dysfunction occurs following previous episodes of deep vein thrombosis or due to age or occupation (long periods of standing). Venous ulceration may often be due to a previous deep vein thrombosis. Preventative measures are aspirin (not indicated for those on warfarin or at risk of stomach ulceration) and other anti-thrombotic drugs, or through the use of anti-embolism hosiery when immobile in hospital, on long-haul air flights or long journeys. Care should be taken not to use any compression garments on patients with arterial disease. Exercise is an important issue in prevention but not always achievable by immobile patients or passengers on a long-haul flight.

Deep-partial thickness burn A deep burn, in which the dermis has been destroyed. The area tends to be anaesthetic as the pain receptors are destroyed. Often white in colour.

Defensive materials Blood cells and fluid — leucocytes, macrophages, etc. These systems react to chemical messengers, immediately following an injury. Their role is to mimic a clinical infection: to establish the means to fight infection before it occurs.

Deglove The epidermis is torn away, exposing the dermis or lower structures. Skin is stripped through trauma. Degloving often occurs in patients who have received long-term steroid therapy.

Degloving injury (SEE Deglove).

Degranulate A number of cell types including neutrophils and mast cells contain granules. These are released from the cell following injury, and are important in inflammation and repair. Granules may be released at a site of trauma, in response to a biochemical stimulus. Mast cell granules contain histamine and serotonin. (SEE Mast cell.)

Dehiscence Separation of the opposed edges of a surgical wound. Usually arises between the sixth and eighth postoperative day. The degree of separation may be partial or complete, with joints or viscera exposed; frequently the consequence of obesity and wound infection.

Demarcation line A distinct line that separates two areas, eg. a sensitivity caused by a dressing would have a redness with a straight demarcation line the same size and shape as the dressing. The tissue beyond the dressing would be normal colour. Cellulitis has an indistinct line between the reddened area and the unaffected area.

Dermatome The instrument used to harvest skin for grafting from a donor site.

Denatured A topical preparation may become altered when in the presence of organic tissue (usually refers to proteins) and lose its efficacy, eg. weak iodine solution and tissue exudate.

Dental alginate Dental alginate is used to form impressions of the teeth. It can also be used in wound assessment, as the dental alginate can be placed into a wound and will set to the size and shape of the wound. The cast can be measured with water displacement, weight or tape measurement of the circumference to give area and volume. This method is not practical unless used by experienced personnel in research.

Dermatosis pl. dermatoses. A generic term for disease/diseases of the skin.

Dermis The dermis is the tough and elastic lower and viable layer of the skin and is composed of collagen fibres interlaced with elastic fibres, both of which give skin its tensile strength. The fibres are held within the dermal matrix, a watery-gel structure. The dermis also contains arterioles, capillaries, sweat glands, sebaceous glands and hair follicles. Nerve endings sensitive to touch, pressure, pain and temperature are widely distributed in the dermis.

Dermo-epidermal junction (DEJ) Basement membrane between dermis and epidermis.

De-roof A blister separates the dermis from the epidermis and the area fills with fluid (SEE Blisters). Removing the blister roof (the epidermis) is named 'de-roofing'.

Deslough Slough may delay wound healing and should be debrided. Many moist dressings are capable of promoting autolysis. (SEE Slough.)

Desiccated Dried out.

Desiccation Drying out.

Destructive phase This phase of wound healing can last from one to seven days, when polymorphs and macrophages are responsible for removing bacteria and devitalised tissue.

Devitalised tissue Tissue that is no longer viable.

Diabetes mellitus A multisystem disorder characterised by relative or absolute lack of insulin leading to uncontrolled carbohydrate metabolism. In 1995, there were more than 130 million people world-wide with diabetes and it is estimated that these figures will increase to 300 million by 2025. Type 1, IDDM (Insulin Dependent Diabetes) and Type 2, NIDDM (Non-Insulin Dependent Diabetes) both cause similar and equally severe complications such as, neuropathy, nephropathy, and retinopathy. Diabetes is associated with impaired wound healing and an increased potential for clinical infection rates.

Diabetic neuropathy Is lack of sensation because of nerve damage. The pathogenesis of neuropathy is multifactorial and includes microvascular disease which leads to nerve degeneration. Hyperglycaemia affects nerve cell mitochondrial function. Defects in the myo-inositol, glutathione and related pathways may also be important. Neuropathy is the commonest complication of diabetes and usually arises within five years of the onset of the disease. Patients with diabetic foot ulceration on the plantar, medial and lateral surfaces will almost all have clinically significant peripheral neuropathy. Generally, there is an adequate blood supply but foot ulceration develops due to high pressures from tight-fitting shoes, or an unnoticed injury

from treading on a nail or pin. Neuropathy can lead to the development of a Charcot joint, a function of neuropathy, osteoporosis and sometimes trauma. (SEE Charcot joint.)

Diapedesis The movement of white cells. Neutrophils adhere to the vascular endothelium and to each other and then move between the junctions of the endothelial cell junctions.

Disinfectant Disinfectants are used as antibacterial agents to destroy bacteria on surfaces. (Antiseptics are used as an antibacterial agent in living tissue.)

Dispersion therapy Where a dressing is used to move fluid from the wound bed and into the dressing. Once in the dressing, the fluid is again dispersed throughout the dressing centre. Generally, these dressings have a high moisture vapour transfer rate. (SEE MVTR.)

Distal Furthest position from the heart.

Donor site A skin graft requires tissue to be harvested from another site on the body — this is a donor site.

Doppler ultrasound Hand-held Doppler ultrasound probe usually contains two piezoelectric crystals, one of which acts as a transmitter of the ultrasonic wave while the other receives the reflected signals. Used for assessment of arterial disease (*Figure 1*). (SEE Ankle brachial pressure index.)

Dorsal Posterior or back of organ or body.

Dorsalis pedis Dorsalis pedis is the continuation of the anterior tibial artery. It can be palpated in the 'V' found in the centre line between the lateral and medial malleoli. It is one of the pulse areas used for Doppler ultrasound examination.

Drain Any means for draining fluid from a sinus or wound. Drains may consist of tubing, a capillary dressing or a wound drainage bag.

Drug tariff A regulatory body that controls all drugs and dressings that are available on prescription. Reimbursement can only occur if the dressing is one of those recommended by the regulatory body and therefore, on the drug tariff. Applies to the UK only, other European countries have equivalent systems.

Dry gangrene Dry gangrene is less likely to produce clinical infection than wet gangrene (SEE Gangrene). A digit with dry gangrene may mummify (SEE Mummify) and will naturally amputate (*Figure 8*).

Dynamic Implies movement. Cells of air mattress or cushion inflate and deflate alternately. The aim of a dynamic mattress is to frequently remove pressure along the length of the body.

Dynamic air mattress (SEE Alternating air mattress).

Dynamic air overlay A slimmer type of alternating mattress which is placed over the original mattress and should not come into contact with the bed base. Used for prevention of pressure ulcers in medium to high-risk patients.

Dysplasia Abnormality in development, in pathology, size, shape, and organisation of cells.

E

Eczema The literal Greek meaning of eczema is to 'boil over'. In eczema, the blood vessels dilate causing erythema and an infiltration of inflammatory cells occurs causing oedema of the dermis and epidermis, thereby causing malfunction of epidermal cells. There is a resultant pruritus, excoriation and lichenification.

Effector molecules (SEE Chemokines).

Efficacy A measure of whether a treatment or intervention produces the desired effect.

Elastic bandage A bandage with extensibility that is generally achieved through latex within the bandage.

Elastin Elastin is the fibrous elastic protein in connective tissues that provides flexibility and elasticity.

Elbow ulcer These painful ulcers are often caused by the patient sitting in a chair with their arms supported by the hard wooden arms. Sometimes due to the patient lifting himself or herself up in bed by pushing their elbows into the mattress, thereby increasing friction and shear forces.

Emollients A mixture of water with a suspension of oil usually with emulsifiers and preservative, some of which can cause allergic reactions. Used to moisturise skin. Can be applied to the bath water or may be used in the form of a cream to soften hard and/or dry skin.

Endogenous Something that is produced or originates within an organism.

Endogenous infection Infection caused by an infectious agent already present in the body, the previous infection having been inapparent.

Endorphin A morphine-like peptide naturally produced by the body in response to neurotransmitters when experiencing extreme stress, fear or pain.

Endothelial tissue A single layer of squamous epithelial cells which lines the cavities of the heart, blood vessels, lymphatics and the serous cavities of the body. Endothelial cells play an important role in inflammation as, in the early phase, they regulate extravasation of plasma, cells and platelets.

Endothelial-derived relaxing factor A vasodilator.

Endothelin A vasoconstrictor.

Endotoxins Toxins produced by bacteria which remain within their structure until they are released on destruction of the bacteria.

Entonox A mixture of nitrous oxide gas and air that provides analgesia and a feeling of well being. Used as an analgesia, for patients with extremely painful wounds at dressing change.

Environmental flora Micro-organisms found in the environment.

Enzyme Enzymes are catalytic proteins that induce chemical changes in other substances.

Enzymatic Relating to an enzyme. Larvae produce enzymes to assist with the digestion of necrotic tissue. Streptokinase and streptodornase are two enzymes that catalyse a breakdown process in necrotic wounds. (SEE Enzymatic debridement.)

Enzymatic debridement An enzymatic dressing, eg. *Varidase* which consists of the enzymes streptodornase and streptokinase; is thought to assist with debridement. Streptokinase has a thrombolytic action, which acts on a substrate of fibrin by activating a fibrinolytic enzyme in human serum and breaks up thrombi. Streptodornase liquefies the viscous nucleoprotein of dead cells or pus. Generally used to rehydrate necrotic wounds. The hardened eschar can be scored prior to applying an enzyme dressing (*Figure 9*). This facilitates effortless access to lower tissue.

Epidermis The epidermis is the outer layer of the skin, sited above the dermis and forms the primary barrier to the body from invading organisms. It is composed of several layers, each of which undergo changes during the process of keratinisation to form the outer most layer, the stratum corneum, or horny layer. This layer consists of flat, non-nucleated, dead cells, which have been keratinised, forming a tough, waterproof protective layer that prevents drying of viable cells. The base layer of the epidermis (germinative layer) is attached to the dermis and receives no blood supply. Basal cells receive nutrients and oxygen by diffusion. Hairs, sweat ducts and sebaceous glands pass from the dermis through the epidermis to reach the surface.

Epidermolysis Splitting and separation of the epidermis from underlying structures, usually accompanied by inflammation, often with signs of blistering. Associated with a disfiguring disease, Epidermolysis bullosa.

Epithelial tissue The cellular lining of the internal and external surfaces of the body including cavities and blood vessels. It comprises specific cell types such as the keratinocyte in the epidermis. The important end stage to wound healing is the growth of surface epithelium, re-epithelialisation. This tissue is programmed to cover a wound as it heals and can do this in two ways:

1. Caterpillar motion — where cells grow behind and push the front cells forward over the wound surface.
2. Leapfrog motion — where a cell migrates over the top of cells and then provides a base for other cells to climb over. While the epithelial tissue is migrating over the surface of the wound, the wound edges are contracting and providing a smaller area for coverage with epithelial tissue.

Epithelialisation When a wound bed has completed proliferation and is level with the surface, epithelial tissue will begin to migrate over the wound. The results are a pink/pale mauve coloured tissue that is fragile and may require protection while it is established (*Figure 10*). (SEE Epithelial tissue.)

Epithelialising (SEE Epithelialisation).

Epithelium (SEE Epithelial tissue).

Erysipelas Commonly caused by *Streptococci* — an infectious condition of the skin or subcutaneous tissue, which usually affects the leg (cellulitis). Can be controlled with antibiotics.

Erythema Redness, as seen in inflammation surrounding wounds, or in areas where prolonged pressure has occluded the local blood supply resulting in inflammatory changes.

Erythrocyte Red blood cell.

Eschar Hard necrotic tissue found generally in pressure ulcers. The tissue has been occluded of blood and dies. It then dehydrates and becomes eschar. This eschar is black and often 'wood' hard. Requires debridement before healing can commence.

EUSOL Edinburgh University Solution of Lime, a hypochlorite solution. Can be painful following application. Not recommended in modern wound care as research illustrates that there are more appropriate and easily obtained dressings which have greater clinical effectiveness. There is also some question of whether there is systemic absorption and how that affects body organs.

Exacerbation An increase in signs or symptoms of disease or pathology. Increased severity.

Excoriated Where the skin has been traumatised — worn away or abraded. Often occurs in the presence of maceration, and can be due to incontinence or inappropriate dressings which cause wetness around the wound margins (*Figure 11*).

Excoriation (SEE Excoriated).

Exogenous External in origin.

Exogenous bacteria Bacteria present in the environment, on curtains, hands, floors, doctors' and nurses' hands and clothes.

Exostosis An abnormal bony outgrowth, generally benign.

Exotoxin Toxins secreted by and found outside bacteria but within the host (infected) cell.

Extracellular matrix (ECM) The so-called non-cellular 'ground substance' of the connective tissue of the dermis. Consists of water, glycosaminoglycans (eg. hyaluronic acid), proteins such as collagen and elastin, fibrinectin, vitro-nectin, and laminin. May be mineralised as in bone or totally fibrous as in tendon. The ECM can influence the behaviour of cells.

Extravasation The leakage of solutions into subcutaneous tissues through intra-venous administration of drugs or fluids can cause minor inflammation or major life threatening damage to the tissues with clinical infection (*Figure 12*).

Extrinsic External in origin. Outside the body.

Exudate Serous fluid that has passed through the walls of a damaged or overextended vein. Often contains growth factors when a wound is acute. May contain bacteria, dead white cells, etc when the wound is chronic. Exacerbated when oedema or hydrostatic pressure is present. Bacteria indirectly causes vaso permeability and this results in increased exudate production. Exudate varies from a thin watery fluid to a thick tenacious fluid, depending upon the condition of the wound. Some exudate is necessary for a moist wound environment.

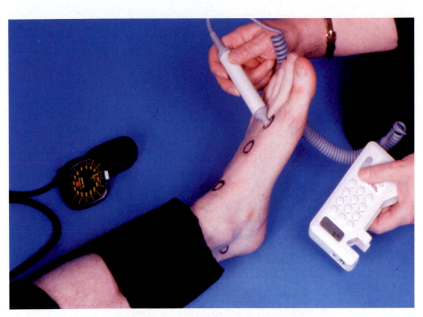

Figure 1: Doppler ultrasound

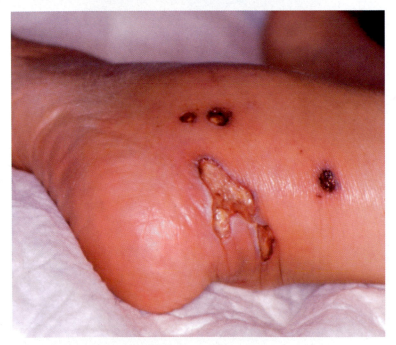

Figure 2: Vasculitis and ulceration

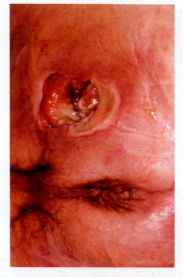

Figure 3: Pressure sore from seating

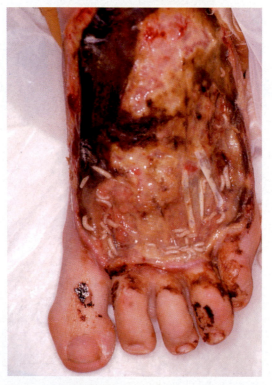

Figure 4: Larvae therapy

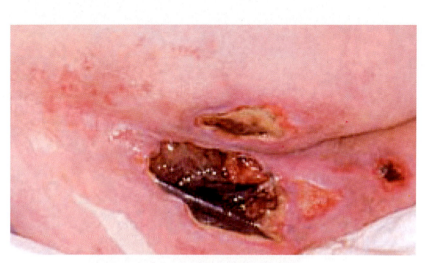

Figure 5: Black wound

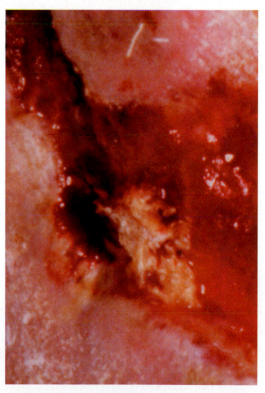

Figure 6: Bone-like calcification growing within a
chronic and long-standing wound

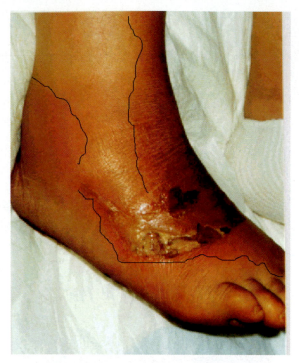

Figure 7: Infected burn

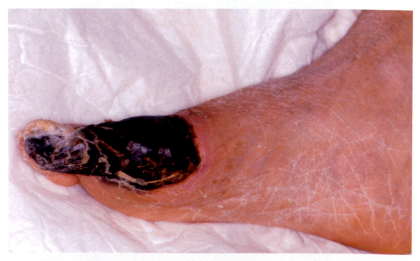

Figure 8: Dry gangrene that has led to mummification

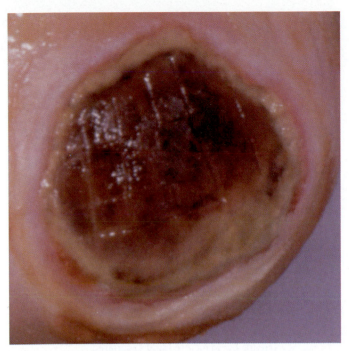

Figure 9: Enzymatic debridement

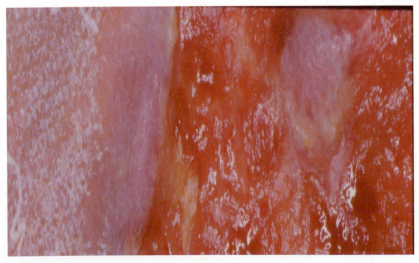

Figure 10: Epithelialisation

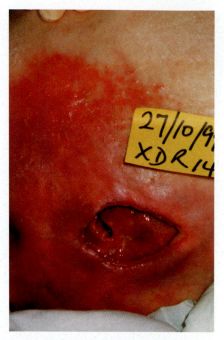

Figure 11: Macerated and excoriated

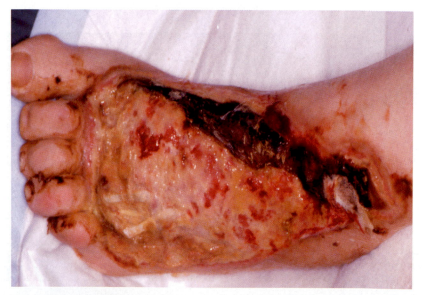

Figure 12: Extravasation

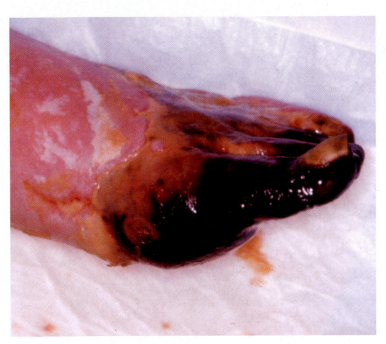

Figure 13: Gangrenous toe

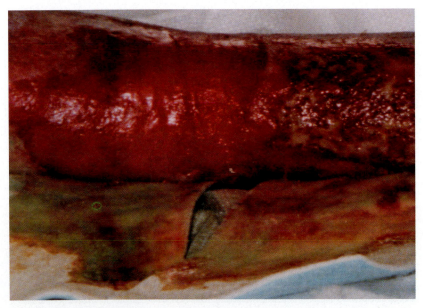

Figure 14: Green wound

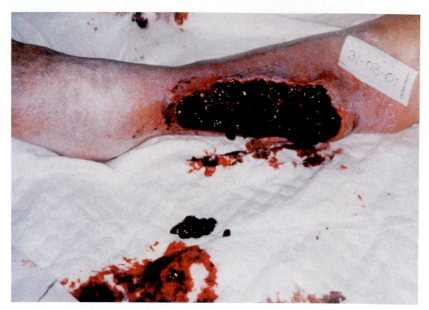

Figure 15: Haematoma

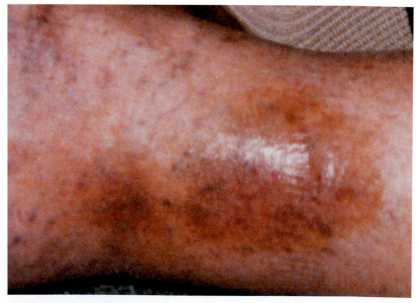

Figure 16: Haemosiderin

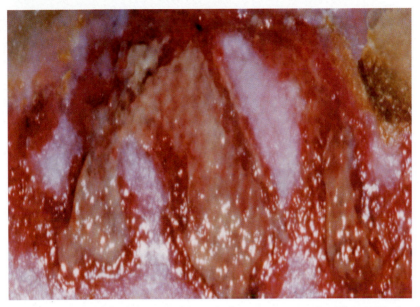

Figure 17: Tissue from a hair follicle which grows outward to form islands of epithelial tissue in the centre of leg ulcers

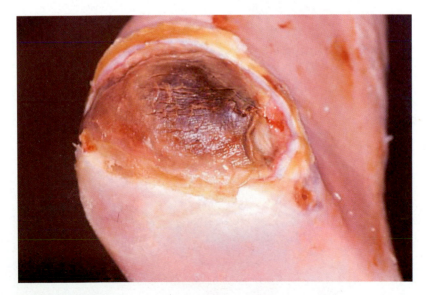

Figure 18: Heel sore

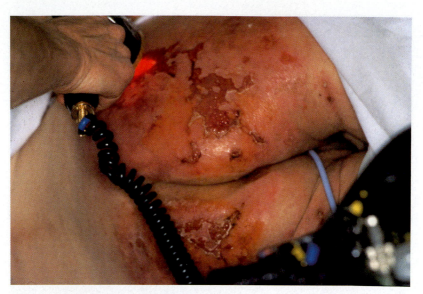

Figure 19: Laser in wound care

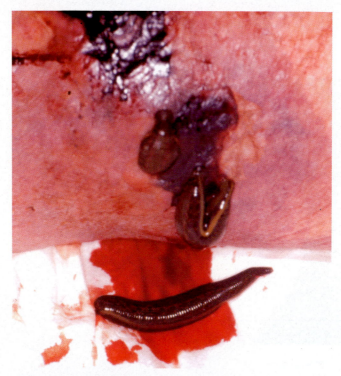

Figure 20: Leech therapy

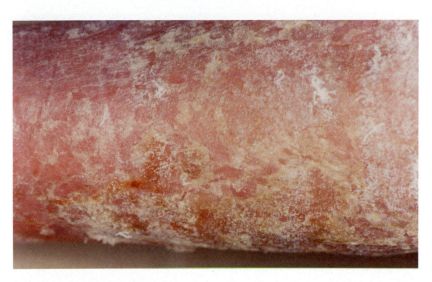

Figure 21: Lipodermatosclerosis

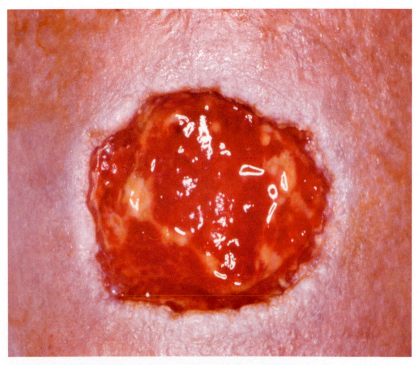

Figure 22: Leg ulceration as a result of liver failure oedema

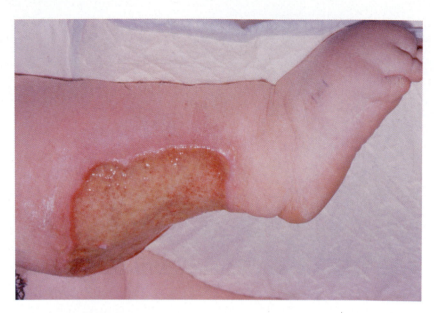

Figure 23: Lymphoedema

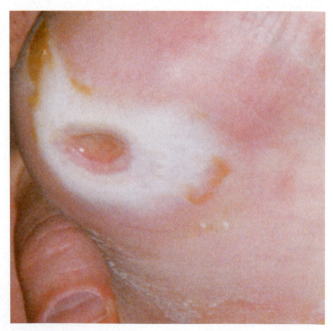

Figure 24: Maceration

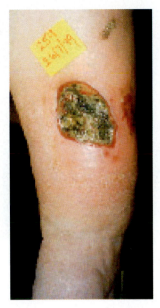

Figure 25: Martorell's ulcer

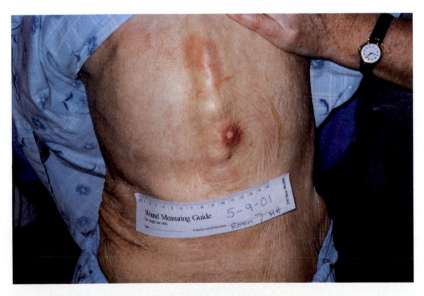

Figure 26: Erythema with necrosis and a 'halo' of inflammation

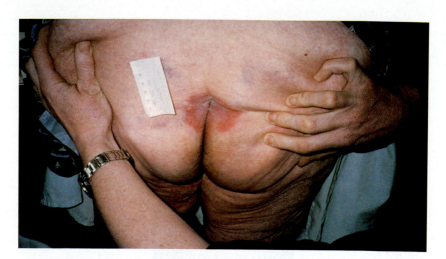

Figure 27: Non-blanching hyperaemia

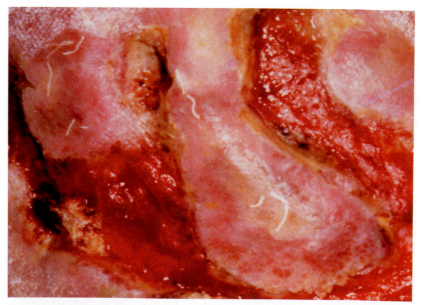

Figure 28: Pink wound

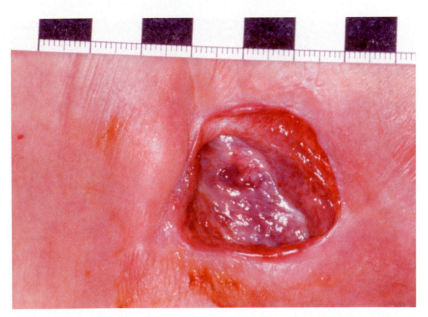

Figure 29: Red wound

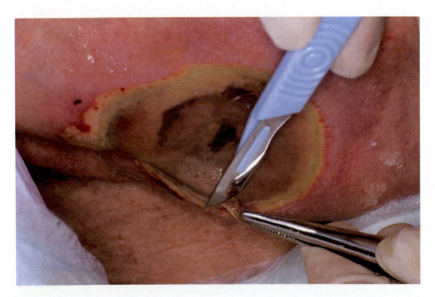

Figure 30: Sharp debridement

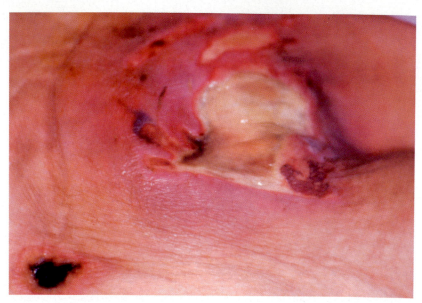

Figure 31: Yellow wound

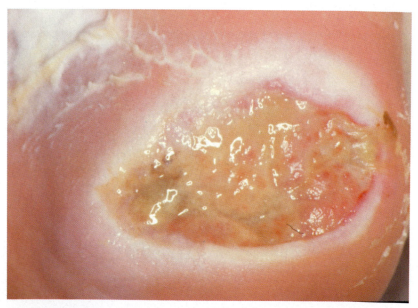

Figure 32: Sloughy wound (yellow wound)

F

Factitious wounds Wounds caused by self-wounding. Often the most difficult to prevent as the psychological motive for the action is not always obvious.

Familial No direct inheritance, but occurs in different members of the same family. Venous ulceration and breast tumours may fall into this category.

Fascia Connective tissue encapsulating (surrounding) organs or muscles.

Fatty acids Naturally occurring long-chain carboxylic acids found in all animal cells. In some infected wounds certain fatty acids and their breakdown products are responsible for malodour.

Femoral artery The main artery of the thigh, a continuation of the external iliac artery.

Fibre filled overlay A mattress overlay that is filled with fibre. Can be used for patients with a low risk for pressure ulcer formation. Washing and use can flatten the fibres and reduce pressure redistribution. A study undertaken by the Medical Devices Agency demonstrated that these overlays might only have a pressure ulcer prevention life of six months.

Fibrin cuff theory This is an unproven theory and is one of many theories of venous leg ulcer formation. The increased pressure of venous hypertension within deep veins creates a back pressure and produces changes in the capillaries. Fibrinogen is one of the molecules to leak into the interstitial fluid. These small molecules unite to form insoluble fibrin which is deposited around capillaries. This 'cuff' prevents diffusion of oxygen and nutrients to the tissues and removal of metabolic wastes.

Fibrin filaments A network of insoluble protein formed from fibrinogen by the action of thrombin during blood clotting. The fibrin filament network forms the essential part of the blood clot.

Fibroblast Cells are responsible for most collagen and elastin synthesis and have a large role to play in wound healing. Their numbers increase when wounds are present and they respond to chemotactic stimuli. Fibroblasts stimulate cell migration, angiogenesis, embryonic development, wound healing and are involved in soft tissue growth and regeneration.

Fibroblast growth factor (FGF) Acidic fibroblast growth factor (alpha FGF) and basic FGF (beta FGF) are two members of a family of structurally related growth factors for dermal cells.

Fibrosis Fibrous tissue formation. Found in scar tissue or as a result of wound inflammation, often with soft tissue adhesions between tissues which can pull, tug and may be uncomfortable. A consequence of injury, characterised by an accumulation of excess collagen. Results in destruction of normal tissue architecture and function. Thought to be stimulated by Transforming Growth Factor ß (TGF).

Fibrous tissue Tissue formed from fibre structures.

Fifty/Fifty (50/50 ointment) An ointment made from 50% paraffin and 50% petroleum jelly. Used to moisten sound skin of patients with leg ulcers.

Filaments Structures that are minute and have the appearance of threads.

Film dressings A transparent film that can be used as a primary dressing in superficial wounds or as a secondary dressing to help to maintain moisture at the wound interface. There are many types of film dressings in the form of sheets, sprays and wipe on films. Some sprays and 'wipe on' films can contain alcohol and this leads to pain when applied. Other 'wipe on' films are painless. Spray on and 'wipe on' films are useful for the protection of peri-wound areas in the prevention of maceration. Sheet films are vapour permeable and permit some evaporation from the wound.

Fissure Split in the skin, may be moist or dry, small or extensive.

Fist test A subjective test to demonstrate the condition of foam mattresses. The hands are linked as a fist and the arms held straight. The assessor leans all the body weight onto the foam. If the assessor feels the bed-base through the foam, it is considered to be 'bottomed out' and requires replacement. This is not an accurate test, particularly for visco-elastic foams.

Fistula A fistula is a passage that has formed between two organs, ie. the bowel and the skin. The opening can leak body fluids such as faeces, bile or urine. Generally difficult to heal as the internal passageway would need to seal prior to surface wound closure.

Fixed ankle joint The foot cannot be flexed or extended. This has implications on the calf muscle pump which requires the calf muscle to contract; a difficult movement with a fixed ankle joint.

Flexed Pertains to a joint. Bending or decreasing the angle between two bones, eg. the foot needs to be flexed when applying compression bandaging.

Flora General term for common microbes on or within the body, or in the environment.

Fluidised bed A large bed containing glass beads with the appearance of fine sand. Air is passed through the beads and the patient is supported by the air-fluidised beads within the bed. Fluid (wound or urine) can be absorbed by the bed and is held until cleaned. Useful for patients with painful skin conditions or burns.

Force Push or pull — energy applied to mobilise or change direction of an object. Can be related to altering the size or shape of an object. Usually measured in Newtons.

Forceps The use of forceps for cleansing wounds in aseptic procedures is no longer recommended as the hardness of the forceps and the mechanical action can damage newly forming tissue. Use of either irrigation or gloved fingers is now the chosen method of cleansing wounds.

Four-layer bandage Four-layer bandaging is the utilisation of four different types of bandages to produce graduated compression for treatment of venous leg ulcers. The four layers consist of an ortho-paedic wool layer, a crepe layer, a long-stretch bandage layer and a cohesive layer. The amount of orthopaedic wool used may vary according to the size and shape of the leg that is to be bandaged. As different size legs require different amounts or types of bandages, four-layer is likely to be called multi-layer.

Fournier's gangrene An acute gan-grenous infection of the scrotum, penis, or perineum involving Gram-positive organisms, enteric bacilli, and anaerobes, which occurs following local trauma, operative procedures, an underlying urinary tract disease, or a distant acute inflammatory process.

Fracture blister A collection of serum, which separates the epidermis from the dermis. Commonly found following ortho-paedic surgery.

Free radicals Free radicals are unpaired electrons in atoms or molecules and, as such, are chemically unstable. They can cause a chain reaction, which is destructive to macromolecules. Chemically very reactive substances released by cells as part of inflammatory and immune responses.

Friable Easily damaged. A wound easily bleeds when touched. Crumbly. As in friable granulation tissue which bleeds on mild trauma.

Friction The resistance of one surface to another that moves over it. The skin and a surface rub together and at the point of contact the skin may be damaged. Friction may be increased by moisture, such as perspiration or urine. It is a contributing factor in the formation of pressure ulcers. Superficial 'rubbing' creates warmth and, in excess, can cause blistering.

Frontal Refers to the front aspect of the body — one of the body planes.

Full-thickness burn Destruction of the dermis and lower structures. Minimal or no pain as the nerve ends are destroyed. White, red or grey in appearance.

Fungating tumour Tumour infiltration into the skin forming a raised exudating fungus-like growth which grows rapidly. A fungating tumour often has a 'cauliflower' appearance and the wound has little vascularity. Therefore, there is a high potential for fungating wounds to contain necrotic tissue and associated anaerobic bacteria. The tumour can invade major arteries and haemorrhage may be a consequence.

Fungating wound A skin lesion, generally malodorous and heavily exuding, that arises from underlying tumours such as those of the breast and histiocytoma. (SEE Fungating tumour.)

Fungicide Substance given to destroy fungal infection of the body.

G

Gait Walking.

Gaiter area That area of the lower limb in which most leg ulcers arise. Named after a garment worn (often in the forces) around the ankle to hold the legs of trousers. The gaiter has a butterfly appearance with the wings of the 'butterfly' over the malleoli.

Gamgee Highly absorbent dressing made of cotton wool with a gauze covering. Used since its invention in the middle 1800s. The inventor (Gamgee) wished to find a dressing that would have an increased capacity for holding fluid. Today, it is only used as a secondary dressing as cotton wool fibres can be shed in the wound and may compromise wound healing.

Gangrene Devitilised 'dead' tissue, caused by failure of the blood supply. May appear dry, wet or be associated with infection by *Clostridium welchii* an anaerobe. (SEE Gas gangrene.) This failure can occur for many reasons. The most common reasons are sustained periods of pressure on a bony prominence and arterial disease with resultant arterial insufficiency to the lower limbs. Dry gangrene in toes leads to mummification of the digit and natural amputation. If the gangrenous toe (*Figure 13*) is moistened through the use of debridement techniques, it will create malodour and open the viable tissue to clinical infection. It is wise to allow dry gangrene to desiccate. Pressure ulcers must always be treated by removing the pressure, and arterial insufficiency should always be referred for vascular assessment.

Gas gangrene A severe form of gangrene caused by anaerobic infection, particularly *Clostridium welchii*. Anaerobic bacteria do not survive easily in an oxygen environment so the odour is lessened once the wound has been debrided and exposed to the air. The onset of gas gangrene is sudden and dramatic. There is a painful tissue swelling due to the build up of gas. When the swollen area is pressed with the fingers crepitus may be detected. Systemic symptoms can develop in the infection and, if untreated, the patient can develop renal failure leading to coma and death.

Gaseous exchange The exchange of oxygen and carbon dioxide that occurs across vascular membranes. Dressings can influence gaseous exchange with wounds. Occlusive dressings are thought to encourage angiogenesis.

Gauze An open weave material often produced from cotton although synthetic products are available. The fabric is absorbent and is a common component of traditional dressings. Used in America for 'wet to dry' debridement as the gauze is soaked in saline and allowed to dry on the wound. It is then torn out to remove any necrotic tissue. This would produce an inflammatory effect within the wound and could initiate wound healing (although the repeated trauma may delay healing). In the UK, gauze is rarely used in chronic wound care because of poor exudate management, lack of bacterial barrier, pain and trauma upon removal, and delayed healing due to fibres left in the wound. Cotton gauze can have a detrimental effect on wounds for a number of reasons, eg:

1. It may shed fibres into the wound and give a foci for infection.
2. The weave of the gauze permits the newly forming capillaries to loop through the holes, so when the dressing is removed, the capillaries are destroyed.

Gel In the wound care context this is a substance which has a high water content in a polymer matrix. Gels are used topically to hydrate dry wounds (or, as specific ultrasound gel to facilitate Doppler assessment).

Gentian violet or crystal violet A dye used as an antiseptic. Known to be carcinogenic. No longer used in wound care.

Germ General and common name for microbes.

Gland Collection of specialised cells that secrete specific substances when stimulated.

Glomus tumour An unusual, benign and very painful, small (around 2mm diameter) vascular growth in the skin or under nail, appears reddish-brown/black.

Glycaemia Glucose in the blood.

Glycoprotein matrix One of the substances found in dermal matrix.

Graduated compression A method of re-establishing blood return to the heart in venous insufficiency. Compression applied at the ankle is high but as the bandage or stocking is applied over the calf and towards the knee, the pressure is gradually reduced. The graduation or reduction is achieved by applying a specialised compression bandage, under constant tension, from toe to knee. (SEE Laplace's law.) The natural shape of the leg is thin at the ankles and wider at the knee. Because of this shape, the constant tension applied will provide graduated compression with higher pressures found at the ankle than at the knee. Types of compression are; compression hosiery, multi-layer (four-layer), short-stretch and long-stretch bandages.

Gram-negative Bacteria which do not take up Gram-stain. Examples are *Pseudomonas aeruginosa,* E. coli and Klebsiella spp. (SEE Gram-staining.)

Gram-positive Bacteria which take up Gram-stain. Examples are *Staphylococcus aureus* and *Streptococci* (Strep. pyogenes). (SEE Gram-staining.)

Gram-staining Gram-staining is a standard laboratory test that distinguishes between the different types of bacteria. The bacteria are stained and those that retain the dye are Gram-positive and those that lose the dye are Gram-negative.

Granulation A complex combination of newly-formed vascular tissues (endothelial cells) and fibroblasts which lay down a matrix of cellular tissues during wound healing. Granulation tissue is the growth of new tissue formed within the collagen matrix in a wound that is left to heal by secondary intention. The appearance will be a deep pink base with red 'lumps' over the surface. These lumps are capillaries that have grown through the wound matrix and have united in loops to give the wound bed the appearance of granules, hence the name granulation tissue. When granulation tissue is apparent, the wound is healing successfully and requires a dressing that will offer protection.

Granuloma Term used to refer to a tumour, benign or malignant, formed from granulation tissue, which may or may not have an epithelial covering.

Greater trochanter A large bony prominence located on the lateral aspect of the femur, just below the neck of the femur. It is often the site for pressure ulcer development due to poor sitting posture, such as a pelvic obliquity (SEE Pelvic obliquity), or sitting in a seat which is too narrow. Damage to the tissue surrounding the greater trochanters is also associated with prolonged side lying.

Green wound The stage of healing or non-healing is sometimes identified through wound colour. This is a subjective method and is not accurate but can be helpful in noting wound changes during assessment and documentation. A green wound is often erroneously referred to as an 'infected' wound. The green colour (*Figure 14*) is the breakdown of *Pseudomonas* — a bacteria that is a strong coloniser, which does not always infect. *Pseudomonas* respond well to silver dressings. (SEE Red wound, Yellow wound, Black wound, Pink wound.)

Growth factors Are a subclass of cytokines, discovered in the late 1970s, and refer to an assortment of small, naturally occurring proteins (peptides) which are thought to direct a variety of biological processes including embryological development, tumour growth and wound repair. Growth factors appear to play a central role among the messengers of the complex process of wound repair and more than 20 types have been identified. Factors recognised in the wound healing process are Platelet Derived Growth Factors, Transforming Growth Factor β, Fibroblast Growth Factors, Human Growth Hormone and Keratinocyte Growth Factor. Generally, a growth factor must bind to a specific cell receptor before it can initiate the required physiological activity. The importance of growth factors in wound healing is now recognised and new dressings incorporate growth factors to try to redress the balance in a non-healing wound.

Guluronic acid Some alginate dressings contain guluronic acid, which maintains its structure — making removal, in one piece, easy. Other alginates contain mannuronic acid, which gives the dressing less form and requires irrigation with normal saline for removal from the wound. (SEE Mannuronic acid.)

H

Haematoma A bruise or collection of blood in the tissues (*Figure 15*). A heparin-based ointment (Lasonil) can be used to reduce bruising and, leeches may be used to stimulate the blood supply into the area, facilitating removal of old blood.

Haemoglobin The pigment that produces the red colour of blood. It is made up of a protein containing the iron containing pigment, haematin or haem. The main function of haemoglobin is to act as a carrier of oxygen.

Haemosiderin Brown with a tinge of red discolouration in skin due to iron deposition within the skin, often associated with venous hypertension and sometimes with a past history of trauma, eg. bruising. In the presence of venous incompetence, hydrostatic pressure occurs and this will stretch the lumen of the veins. This increased pressure forms gaps between the vascular wall, which allows fluid to leak into the tissues, resulting in oedema. The stretching of capillary lumen allows leakage of plasma proteins, plasma, and red blood cells into the tissue, and this causes pigmentation of the skin leaving a brown stain (haemosiderin). This is a permanent mark (*Figure 16*).

Haemosiderosis The condition where there is haemosiderin (iron) deposition in the skin.

Haemostasis The control of bleeding — preventing bleeding. Method of reducing or stopping blood flow from a damaged blood vessel.

Haemostat The means by which bleeding is controlled. For example, calcium alginate wound dressing, silver sulphadiazine, used to arrest bleeding from acute and chronic wounds.

Hair follicles Pockets of skin from which a hair will grow. The follicle is completely invaginated by epithelial tissue and it is the tissue from the hair follicle that will grow outward to form islands of epithelial tissue in the centre of leg ulcers (*Figure 17*). Collection of cells within the dermis which produce hair, usually have a sebaceous gland as part of the complex.

Halo A ring of inflammation surrounding a site may be referred to as an inflammatory halo.

Hammocking A term used to describe a situation where the cover of a mattress or cushion is stretched so tightly over the inner material that the user is unable to gain contact with the internal pressure-reducing materials, thereby reducing the mattress or cushion's ability to prevent pressure ulcers.

The standard King's Fund mattress, used within the health service for many years, had an internal core of foam that was made deliberately larger than the cover. This led to an increased interface pressure between the patient and the mattress and could be referred to as 'hammocking'. Constant wear placed strain on the cover causing it to stretch. The outcome was a dent where the patient would sit. Hammocking can also be caused by material and plastic sheets which are stretched over the mattress and tucked in tightly.

Hamstrings A group of three muscles, namely biceps femoris, semimembranosus and semitendinosus, situated on the posterior aspect of the thigh. They all originate on the ischial tuberosity of the pelvis, with the biceps femoris inserting into the head of the fibula, the semi-membranosus inserting into the medial condyle of the tibia, and the semi-tendinosus inserting into the medial side of the tibia just below the knee. All are responsible for both hip extension and knee flexion. In some instances, particularly due to poor sitting posture or increased muscle tone, the hamstrings may become shortened, and this reduces an individual's ability to achieve an upright sitting position. As a result, the person will often adopt a slouched position or 'posterior pelvic tilt', increasing potential for sacral pressure ulcers.

Hansen's disease Leprosy. Symptoms include neuropathy and ulceration following infection by mycobacterium leprae.

Hartmann's solution An isotonic solution that is sometimes used to re-establish electrolyte balance. Also known as Ringer-Lactate, a physiological electrolyte solution that can be used for wound irrigation.

Heat sensitive foams (SEE Visco-elastic foam).

Heel ulcer Heels may develop pressure ulcers even on the most progressive mattresses. This is due to a variety of contributing factors: patients with poor arterial supply may be wrongly provided anti-embolism stockings (a high risk factor). During the day patients often sit out of bed with their heels on the floor, which places them at extreme high risk. Furthermore, time spent on waiting trolleys or on theatre tables can contribute to heel ulcers. It is also possible that mattresses with low interface pressure under sacral areas may not offer the same low ratio of pressure under heels (*Figure 18*).

Heloma Latin term for hard corn.

Heparin An anticoagulant that occurs naturally and is used clinically as the low molecular weight heparin (LMWH) to prevent clot formation during surgery (Thromboprophylaxis). The action of heparin is to prevent prothrombin conversion to thrombin. The liver naturally produces heparin. Can be injected to prevent deep vein thrombosis or an established thrombosis from growing larger.

Herpes Viral infection, usually of the skin, causing painful vesicular lesions, eg. cold sores are caused by herpes simplex.

High compression In Europe, high compression of 60mmHg can be used in patients with deep vein disease. Not often used within the UK. High compression is achieved through increasing the layers of compression bandages. May refer to bandaging applied firmly to manage the complications (oedema, ulceration) associated with venous incompetence, or may refer to how firmly tissues are squashed in a particular area on loading, eg. sitting, lying, walking.

Histamine A substance that is produced in response to injury or allergy. Released from granules in Mast cells in tissues. An important mediator of the inflammatory reaction. This reaction delivers defences to the site of injury by increasing permeability. Produces the recognised clinical signs of inflammation — redness, swelling and pain.

Holistic assessment In tissue viability, a holistic assessment of a patient is to review all systems and the effect that any noted pathology may have on wound healing or prevention of pressure ulcers. Unless there is bleeding occurring, the last consideration is the wound. A way of assessing and considering the whole person, their situation and other influences on their lifestyle.

Homeostasis The body's natural mechanism for maintaining health constancy (or balance) and ensuring survival. Maintenance of normality within the body, includes blood pressure control, and thermoregulation.

Homogenous Of similar consistency or structure.

Honey Certain forms of honey, for example, Manuka or Leptospermum honey, may be used to aid chronic wound healing. Honey is naturally produced by bees and has been used in wound care for centuries. It has natural antiseptic properties and exerts an osmotic pressure that restricts bacterial proliferation. Honey will soon be licensed for wound care but this does not permit the purchase of any honey for use on wounds. Some honey may contain botulinum toxins and, therefore, must have passed strict safety tests prior to use on open skin. Australia and New Zealand grow a Manuka plant that contains antiseptic properties, and the bees that feed on this plant produce honey that has high antiseptic properties. It is this honey that will soon be licensed for wound care.

Host An organism that is infected with or fed upon by a parasite or pathogen.

Hyaluronic acid (HA) Also known as hyaluronan. Is a major carbohydrate component of the extracellular matrix, is found in most parts of the body and is generally accepted as being associated with wound repair. Wound tissues exhibit an increase in hyaluronic acid in the early stages of wound repair. It is known that foetal wounds heal without scarring and that hyaluronic acid is responsible for this. It is probable that fragments of HA promote angiogenesis by stimulating endothelial cells through binding to ICAM-1. HA also induces cytokine production by macrophages through binding to the CD-44 receptor. Hyaluronan solutions are highly osmotic and can control tissue hydration during periods of change, such as the inflammatory process. When this occurs, the result is facilitation of cell migration and division. The viscous nature of hyaluronan prevents bacteria from reaching the wound tissues.

Hyaluronidase Enzyme which breaks down hyaluronic acid.

Hydrocellular Dressing which holds liquid within its microscopic structure.

Hydrocolloids The components of a major class of moist wound healing dressings. Consist of a mixture of pectin, gelatin, sodium carboxymethyl cellulose and elastomers. Generally presented in a self-adhesive wafer dressing (although it can be found in hydrofibre or paste form). Hydro-colloids are slightly absorbent and provide an occlusive environment for wounds.

Hydrocortisone A steroid hormone produced by adrenal cortex (corticosteroid), used systemically and topically to reduce inflammation.

Hydrofibre dressing A wound dressing, consisting of fibres of hydrocolloid, for example, sodium carboxy-methylcellulose, which absorbs and retains fluid and provides a moist environment.

Hydrogel Hydrogels generally consist of approximately 70% water and some starch. There are some absorptive qualities. Provided in sheets or gels. Hydrogels are an excellent means for rehydrating necrotic wounds. (SEE Amorphous structure.)

Hydrogel sheets The sheets are made up of gelable polysaccharide agarose, cross-linked with polyacrylamide. They are used in wound care to provide a moist wound interface. Some hydrogel sheets are useful in reducing scar tissue.

Hydrogen peroxide Hydrogen perox-ide consists of hydrogen and oxygen. Liberates oxygen on contact with organic material (pus) and this reaction causes the liquid to froth. Used in cleansing of wounds. Some small studies accuse hydrogen peroxide of causing air emboli when placed into a sinus or cavity. Not often used in the UK because the liquid has the potential to damage healing tissues and because of the potential for an air embolus. However, the frothing liquid is useful in accident and emergency centres for contaminated grazes.

Hydrophilic Water loving. Dressings that are hydrophilic will absorb fluid. Foam dressings would be an example.

Hydrophobic Water hating. Dressings that reject water. Paraffin gauze is an example.

Hydropolymers Long chains of a substance incorporating water molecules within their structure.

Hydrostatic Fluid that is still, unmoving. Implies no change in fluid balance, it is in equilibrium.

Hydrostatic pressure Pressures within tissues associated with fluid content and efficiency of blood flow. Fluid collects within the veins due to incompetent valves. The volume of blood collecting in the veins places the veins under pressure causing them to become engorged and dilated. This pressure separates the cell junctions within the veins and this allows the escape of fluid and macromolecules into the tissues.

Hyperaemia Amount of blood in excess of requirements.

Hyperbaric oxygen Deliberately elevated partial pressure of oxygen delivered through a whole body oxygen chamber or through topical hyperbaric therapy. Hyperbaric oxygen elevates the plasma oxygen level in proportion to the partial pressure of inspired oxygen. This enables oxygen to be delivered to the cells even in the absence of haemoglobin, ensuring that the oxygen supply is rich for wound repair and leucocyte activity.

Hyperglycaemia Raised blood glucose level.

Hypergranulation Overgranulation, excessive laying down of new blood vessels creating a bulge of highly vascular tissue which bleeds easily. A wound that has granulation tissue forming that grows beyond the surface level of the wound and prevents epithelialisation from occurring. This phenomenon may occur because of a previous clinical infection that has disturbed the equilibrium of the inflammatory phase or it may occur due to the excellence of modern dressings, which encourage granulation tissue. Reduction of hypergranulation may be achieved through use of any of the following: foam dressings, silver nitrate, double hydrocolloid, hydrocortisone cream, pressure.

Hyperplasia An increase in the number of cells in a tissue or organ. An abnormal state of cell division, usually a response to injury or inflammation.

Hypersensitivity Patients with wounds, particularly those with venous leg ulcers, often exhibit local allergic reactions to treatments. Typically, these reactions are 'sensitisation' or hypersensitivity reactions (delayed hypersensitivity type IV). The usual allergens are excipients in topically applied preparations, such as creams, ointments, pastes, etc, or adhesives in dressings, or rubber in elastic bandages. Immediate hypersensitivity (anaphylactic reactions, cell mediated type I) rarely occur. These manifest most frequently as urticaria and rarely as angio-oedema. Dermatologists justifiably advocate patch testing of patients with leg ulcers.

Hypertensive vein A vein that is engorged to capacity due to reflux of blood through incompetent valves. The raised volume of blood increases hydrostatic pressure.

Hypertrophic scar An enlargement or overgrowth of scar tissue characterised by excessive deposition of collagen. May result from insufficient protein degradation. Hypertrophic scars form within wound boundaries and can regress, whereas keloid scarring extends beyond the wound boundaries and tends to remain elevated. (SEE Keloid scarring.) There are silicone hydrogel dressings to reduce the appearance of scar tissue. Injections of hydrocortisone will assist in reduction. Pressure garments (in burn scarring) may prevent overgrowth or contractures in scar tissue.

Hypertrophy Overgrowth of tissue, particularly an overgrowth in the size of cells that form the tissue. Excess size of a tissue, may be adaptive, eg. of muscle with exercise, or associated with pathological process.

Hypoallergenic Applied to topically-applied agents such as adhesives, cosmetic ingredients, etc, implying very low or no potential to cause sensitisation.

Hypochlorite A bleach. Has been used to deslough wounds, particularly in the form of EUSOL (Edinburgh University Solution of Lime). Not often used today as it is painful, damaging to newly formed tissue and may be absorbed into the system. (SEE EUSOL.)

Hypoglycaemia Low blood glucose level.

Hypoproteinaemia Level of total protein within the blood is abnormally low, often associated with poor nutrient intake or absorption.

Hypovolaemia A reduction in circulating blood due to blood loss or due to the effect of shock. Will delay wound healing.

Hypoxia A lack of oxygen in circulating blood. Can lead to a potential for clinical infection due to low oxygen availability for phagocytes. Hypoxia will also delay wound healing, as the newly forming tissues require oxygen to develop.

I

Iatrogenic Effects of treatment brought about by a (medical) intervention, usually relates to the adverse effects of treatment.

Ideal wound healing environment
(SEE Optimum wound healing environment.)

Idiopathic An abnormal physiological reaction which occurs for unpredicted and unpredictable reasons.

Immunity The body's natural defence against disease or infection.

Impact Sudden loading of tissues by a force or pressure.

Impetigo Skin condition due to *strepto-coccal* infection, painful, bright red, sometimes vesicular spots on affected skin.

Incidence A measurement taken over a given time span, ie. how many pressure ulcers develop in a hospital over a one-week or one-month period.

Incised An incised wound is an injury to the skin caused by a sharp cutting implement, such as a knife, broken glass, or a surgeon's scalpel.

Incompetency Can refer to function of semi-lunar valves in veins.

Infarction Area of ischaemia and perhaps necrosis following marked inhibition or cessation in blood flow. In wounds, infarction is seen as necrotic (black) tissue.

Infection Caused by micro-organisms, which evade the victim's immunological defences, enter and establish themselves within tissues of the potential host and multiply successfully. The following are likely to be present: suppuration, cellulitis, lymphangitis, sepsis, bacteraemia, pyrexia, tachycardia, tachypnoea, raised white cell count. Not to be confused with colonisation or contamination.

Infective necrosis A clinical infection which has led to death of the tissues. Dead tissue with a tendency for the bacterial pathogen to spread.

Infestation An invasion of parasites. The body is invaded, usually by parasites, eg. scabies and lice.

Inflammation The purpose of the inflammation is to defend the tissues against bacterial invasion and, at the same time, deliver mediators to stimulate the wound healing process. It is a complex sequence of events which has yet to be fully understood where, following injury, the classic clinical features of inflammation; redness (erythema), heat (calor), swelling (oedema) and pain arise, sometimes also with loss of function of the part. The redness, swelling, pain and heat is initiated through production of histamine by mast cells. The signs of inflammation can be mistaken for clinical infection, although if the redness and swelling is less than three days, it is unlikely to be infection.

Inflammatory Describes the inflamed state. (SEE Inflammatory response.)

Inflammatory response The physiological response that immediately follows injury, and protects the system against invasion of bacteria. (SEE Inflammation.)

Inhibitor Substance which restrains the effect of another, there may be competitive inhibition between different bacterial colonies where one prevents the other from rampantly spreading.

Intelligent foam (SEE Visco-elastic foam).

Interactive dressing An interactive dressing will mediate changes within the wound bed or wound fluid, eg. iodine, hydro-colloids, etc. This is the opposite to dressings (such as foam dressings) which will absorb exudate but will not alter the status of the wound. The dressing, whether interactive or passive, should be selected according to the individual wound requirements and should offer an ideal wound-healing environment. A colonised or sloughy wound may require an inter-active dressing whereas a healing wound may require a passive dressing.

Intrathoracic pressure During inspir-ation, there is a negative pressure created within the veins. This pressure 'pulls' blood back to the heart from the extremities. This pressure can be heard through a Doppler ultrasound placed over a vein in the arm.

Insufficiency Often refers to blood supply, eg. venous insufficiency, where the veins do not function optimally.

Intercellular Between cells.

Intercellular adhesion molecule (ICAM) A glycoprotein present on cells, it is involved in cell-cell recognition and in the inflammatory process.

Interdigital Between toes and fingers.

Interface pressures (SEE Pressure).

Interleukin A variety of naturally occurring polypeptides that are members of the family of cytokines which effect functions of specific cell types. They are produced by lymphocytes, monocytes and various other cell types and are released by cells in response to antigenic and non-antigenic stimuli. The interleukins, of which there are 12 identified to date, modulate inflammation by regulating growth, mobility and differentiation of cells.

Intermittent claudication A symptom of arterial disease characterised by leg pain and weakness brought on by exercise. The symptom disappears following rest.

Intermittent compression therapy A small compressor to which one or two tubes are connected from the proximal end to one or two inflatable boots. The air is intermittently expelled and then inflated, expanding the boot for a short period of

time. The boots alternate in 'squeezing' or compressing the legs, causing reduction in venous hypertension.

Inter-rater reliability How much variation in measurement there is between different people.

Interstitial The spaces between cells forming the tissue. Within the tissues.

Interstitial fluid The fluid that is found in the spaces between tissue cells. In oedema there is an increased volume.

Interstitial spaces Between organs or planes of other tissues, there may be small gaps that are usually filled with interstitial fluid.

Intertrigo An eczematous and irritating area of skin caused by apposition of two moist surfaces. Skin soreness due to chafing/rubbing of one surface over the other, often associated with yeast infection, eg. candida albicans.

Intracellular Within the cell.

Intrinsic Particular to or contained within a person.

Iodine Solutions and other formulations of iodine have a long history as topical antiseptics in wound care. Iodine is effective against Gram-positive and negative bacteria, anaerobes, viruses, fungi and yeasts. Concerns related to the use of iodine are for systemic absorption and toxicity to newly-formed tissues. Recent developments include 'iodophore' compounds such as povidone iodine (PVP-I) and cadexomer (modified starch hydrogel) iodine; these are sustained delivery compounds which slowly release elemental iodine into the wound. Such compounds are now incorporated into topical wound dressings and preparations and are generally regarded as safe and effective for the debridement and treatment of a variety of colonised and infected wounds. The older formulations such as tinctures and iodoform are no longer recommended for wounds.

As a pre-operative skin preparation, solutions of PVP-I are safe and effective. The use of iodine preparations on open wounds should be avoided in patients with thyroid and renal disorders, children under two years, and those receiving lithium therapy. When iodine is absorbed into the system, it converts to iodide and may be used by the enzyme myeloperoxidase. As myeloperoxidase has an antibacterial element, the utilisation of iodide may be useful in prevention of infection.

Iodine cadexomer An iodine-carbohydrate paste dressing that absorbs exudate and releases iodine over a period of time. The time period relies on the amount of pus to be found within the wound as pus negates the effect of iodine.

Irrigation The use of fluids and solutions to cleanse a wound of debris and other contaminants. Irrigation using normal saline delivered by a 30ml syringe and 18–20-gauge needle is a recommended method of wound cleansing. The solution should be applied at a pressure of 7 pounds per square inch (psi). Lower pressures would merely redistribute the bacteria and debris and greater pressures may drive the bacteria into tissues, thereby potentially causing clinical infection. The practitioner may find difficulty in judging how hard to press the syringe to deliver the recommended amount of pressure. A pressurised canister of saline can provide the required pressure. Before cleansing any wound, the practitioner should assess whether it requires cleansing. If there is little to clean then irrigation could be dangerous to fragile tissues.

Iron deposition (SEE Haemosiderosis).

Ischaemia Localised deficiency of arterial blood. May be due to occlusion of the arteries due to atherosclerosis or may be due to local occlusion of tissues due to pressure and is often acutely painful.

Ischaemic foot May be due to occlusion of the arteries by atherosclerosis or to local occlusion of tissues caused by pressure. The appearance of the foot can be blue, white or dusky pink.

Ischial tuberosities Situated at the base of the ischium of the pelvis, the two ischial tuberosities are rounded bony prominences, which when an individual is in a sitting position, support a large percentage of the body weight. Their shape, and position in relation to the femurs, make them very unstable supporting structures for sitting. Pressure ulcers which are sited on the tuberosities are normally related to sitting or being semi-recumbent in bed.

Island dressing Dressing contains a different material (and therefore function) in its centre.

Islands of epithelium (SEE Hair follicle.) Islands of epithelium that grow outward from the centre of the wound, and have hair follicles as their source: important as focal point for re-epithelialisation in burns. When healing, a wound may show patches of pearly-pink epithelialising skin (*Figure 17*).

Isotonic solution A solution comparable in osmolarity to another. For example, the solution used in a wound is the same osmotic pressure as the fluids within the wound (normal saline 0.9% sodium chloride is isotonic as are Ringer's and Hartmann's solutions).

J

Jelly (SEE Gel).

Jelonet® A paraffin loaded gauze designed to reduce adherence to wound surfaces. May require application of several layers. (SEE Tulle Gras.)

Jobst stocking Jobst compression garments used to reduce hypertrophic scarring after burn injuries. Jobst hosiery provide compression for the treatment of leg ulceration. There is a zip that runs from the ankle to the top of the calf to simplify application.

Joule A unit measuring energy, eg. energy expended in moving a body over a distance.

K

Kallikrein Enzyme found in blood plasma following injury. Causes vaso-dilation.

Keloid scar A scar will continue to mature over a two-year period. Sometimes the scar tissue 'overgrows' and becomes discoloured. This scar is prominent and misshapen and can increase in size. Keloid scarring is characterised by excessive deposition of collagen and may result from insufficient protein degradation. Keloid scarring extends beyond the wound boundaries and tends to remain elevated, whereas hypertrophic scars form within wound boundaries and can regress. (SEE Hypertrophy.)

Keratin Structural fibrous protein which forms the stratum corneum of the epidermis, the most superficial layer of the skin.

Keratinisation The process whereby epidermal cells (keratinocytes) differentiate to form the stratum corneum. The process involves complex biochemical changes including the synthesis of keratin protein, and gross morphological changes.

Keratinocyte A cell type which synthesises keratin. The predominant cell type of the epidermis, which arises from mitosis at the level of the basement membrane and migrates slowly towards the skin surface, differentiating morphologically and bio-chemically into the stratum corneum cell. This is then shed into the environment in an orderly fashion in the process of desquamation.

Keratinocyte growth factor (KGF) Stimulates granulation and believed to exert a proliferative effect on epithelial cells.

Keratosis An abnormal condition of the skin usually with thickening of the epidermis.

Kinin Molecules involved in the inflammation and repair processes.

Knitting needle syndrome Some patients may despair at the idea of their wound healing as the district nurse will no longer visit and this could lead to complete social isolation. It is occasionally suggested that patients may use a knitting needle to reach their wounds to disturb healing. This is anecdotal and unproven.

Koilonychia A spoon-shaped nail, may be indicative of poor central and/or peripheral blood supply and oxygenation.

Kyphosis The anatomical shape of the thoracic spine is slightly concave forward, known as a minimal thoracic kyphosis. In some instances this curvature becomes increased, frequently caused as a result of poor sitting posture and in particular a posterior pelvic tilt. The development of the kyphosis causes the lumbar lordosis to be lost. As the curvature increases, the internal organs are compressed and their function is consequently compromised. The spinous processes of the spine become prominent, and due to the poor sitting posture, increased body weight pushes them against the backrest. Pressure ulcers develop over each process as a result.

L

Laceration A tearing or splitting of the skin caused by blunt trauma, such as a blow from a fist or foot or with a hammer or baseball bat.

Lamina A thin layer in a tissue.

Laminin Protein within the dermis.

Langer's lines The lines of orientation of subcutaneous collagen fibres. These vary in direction with the region of the body surface and its movement. Surgical incisions across these lines are not conducive to healing as stretching tends to open the wound.

Lanolin A derivative of sheep's wool, used as an emollient to hydrate dry or rough skin, can cause contact allergy.

Laplace's law Laplace's law calculates the pressure produced by a compression bandage and dictates higher pressure on a small compressed limb than a large compressed limb. Therefore, pressure will be greater on a thin ankle than on a thick calf. The calculation is achieved by multiplying the tension produced under the bandage by the number of layers and the equal application. This is divided by limb circumference and width of the bandage. (SEE Compression.)

Larvae (SEE Maggots.) In wound debridement the commonly used fly is *Lucilia sericata* (green bottle fly) (*Figure 4*).

Larval therapy Maggots are not a new component in wound care, they have been found in wounds over centuries and have possibly been responsible for saving lives on many battlefields. Bridgend biosurgical research centre are now breeding the green bottle fly and sterilising the eggs for use in wound care throughout the world. These larvae produce powerful proteolytic enzymes that degrade and liquefy necrotic tissue, which they then ingest. Although they digest devitalised tissue, they do not normally harm healthy tissue. Those patients with malodorous and longstanding wounds often welcome this treatment to speed up the healing. The action of the larvae is thought to stimulate wound healing and the maggots eliminate all but one bacterium from the wound (thereby eliminating malodour). Treatment with maggots can be cost effective, as debridement is rapid, although practitioners may find it distasteful to apply. The maggots produce powerful proteolytic enzymes that degrade and liquefy necrotic tissue and can be successful in debriding wounds.

Laser therapy The application of light energy waves over a wound to stimulate the healing process. Low-level laser therapy is used at approximately 10 joules per cm^2 with powers of 50m W. Largely unproven as a treatment. Often applied to wounds by physiotherapists (*Figure 19*).

Lateral On the outer side of the body.

Lateral support Thoracic support attached to a wheelchair or armchair, to provide support to the trunk, thereby preventing the patient from leaning heavily to one side. Correct positioning of thoracic supports may be employed to reduce a flexible compensatory scoliosis.

Laudable pus In the eighteenth century, there was a belief that pus assisted with wound healing. The doctors decided that if a wound did not contain pus, an amount would be taken from another wound and placed into the pus free wound. Due to advances in microbiology, it is now recognised that this would be a dangerous practice if used today.

Lavage Washing of a wound or other area.

Lavender May be used as a topical preparation as a stimulant and possible antimicrobial treatment for wound management, there is currently insufficient data on its action in this area.

Leech The leech is a 32-segmented invertebrate, with each segment containing an elementary brain (*Figure 20*). The leech will seek its prey and fasten to the victim's surface by use of posterior suckers. The leech is used to reduce haematomas, to reduce venous congestion in plastic surgery and to encourage blood flow into poorly perfused areas.

Left ventricular failure (LVF) The left side of the heart ceases to work effectively leading to ascending oedema. As a result, oedematous tissues are poorly supplied with oxygen and nutrients and ulceration may occur. The site of the ulceration can be anywhere affected by ascending oedema. People with LVF should never receive compression therapy without first reducing the oedema as this can flood the system with fluid. In such a situation, the heart would be unable to cope with the increased demand, resulting in a total failure of the system.

Leg club A club for patients who are at risk of ulcer development or have an established leg ulcer. The club is overseen and guided by nurses who recommend and carry out treatment. The clubs are self-funding and directed by the patients who view the club as a social gathering. The club meets weekly and patients sit together, have tea and discuss their symptoms with each other. They are not segregated for treatment and freely share their experiences with each other. This format supports patient empowerment and education. The words 'venous' or 'ulcer' are kept from the title of the club to enable those patients who wish to prevent future or recurrent ulcers to feel free to attend.

Leg ulcer clinic A clinic, usually run by nurses or a multi-disciplinary healthcare team, especially organised for patients with leg ulcers. Patients attend at a pre-determined time and are assessed and treated by a professional. Patients attending leg ulcer clinics tend to have higher healing rates than individuals treated at home.

Lesion Abnormality in tissue, may be seen as tissue injury, sores, ulcers, tumours, cysts or rashes, etc.

Leucocytes White blood cell of which there are three types: Polymorphonuclear (granular) cells, monocytes and lymphocytes (includes eosinophils, neutrophils). Some of these cells are responsible for defence at a time of injury.

Leucocyte chemotaxis The movement of leucocytes to an area of injury in response to chemical messengers.

Ligation Tying up a blood vessel to stop bleeding.

Link-nurse (Also termed Lead nurse.) A qualified nurse takes on responsibility for assessing tissue viability risk for patients in their own ward/community. Also refers to a nurse who takes on the role of link between specialist nurses and the ward or community area. Link-nurses generally assist with education, advice, audit and pressure ulcer prevention.

Lichen planus A persistent skin condition characterised by shiny, flat-topped papules — found mainly on the flexor surfaces of limbs. Cause is unknown and the lesions tend to resolve spontaneously after months or sometimes years.

Lint A fluffy, usually cotton, traditional wound dressing, currently not used owing to problems with development of granulomas around the cotton fibres.

Lipases Enzymes which break down fats.

Lipids A group of fats and fat-like substances characterised by being insoluble in water and soluble insolvents, such as ether, chloroform, and methanol. They contain aliphatic hydrocarbons, for example, fatty acids esterified to glycerol, long-chain bases and carbohydrates. Examples are: phospholipids, vitamin A, and ceramides.

Lipodermatosclerosis A clinical feature of venous leg ulceration. The dermis and superficial adipose tissue become fibrosed and feel hard. Lack of nutrients and diminished oxygen exchange in venous insufficiency, cause an overall deterioration of the tissues and continued deposit of waste products in the tissues. Often the patient has an 'upside down champagne bottle' leg shape (*Figure 21*).

Lipodystrophy Defective fat metabolism leading to progressive loss of fat in tissues.

Lipoedema A chronic, common and infrequently recognised condition causing bilateral enlargement of the legs in women, due to oedema of subcutaneous fat.

Lipoma Benign, fatty tumour which may spontaneously disappear or predispose to ulceration due to increased tissue bulk, which causes pressure and ischaemic effects on adjacent tissues and blood vessels.

Liquefaction Producing liquid from a more solid form, ie. maggots will liquefy necrotic tissue to enable them to suck up the fluid.

Liver failure oedema Manifested as ascities around the abdomen. However, low serum albumin leads to low osmotic pressures and a collection of fluid within the tissues, which results in swollen limbs and potential for leg ulceration (*Figure 22*).

Load A general term for pressure, shear, friction, torsion and tension which may be applied to the skin and deeper tissues.

Local anaesthesia Effect produced by local application of an anaesthetic. Used in injection or cream form to reduce pain of a procedure. (SEE Topical anaesthetic.) The cream is often applied to reduce pain from painful injections. In Europe (and often in hospices in the UK), anaesthetic cream is used to reduce pain in acutely painful wounds. It is not used in this form in the UK, as the products are not licensed for open wounds.

Locomotion Movement from one place to another.

Long-stretch bandages Long-stretch bandages have a true extensibility and stretch greater than 100% of the original length. They are applied at 50% stretch, which requires a skilled and experienced bandager. It is the pressure resulting from compression that encourages venous return. The long-stretch bandage forms part of the multi-layer bandage regime.

Lordosis The shape of the lumbar region of the spine is convex forward, and this is known as a lumbar lordosis. This can become exaggerated as a compensatory posture due to an increased anterior tilt of the pelvis.

Low adherence Dressings with a reduced tendency to stick to the wound surface.

Low air loss mattress A mattress replacement system that has minute holes throughout the surface of the mattress. Air is constantly passed out of the air-holes and into the atmosphere. This equalises the pressure within the mattress — particularly when the patient moves. The interface pressure relies on pressure redistribution (not pressure relief as in dynamic systems).

Lumen The space within a tube such as a blood vessel. In atheroma this tube or lumen will be narrowed.

Lupus erythematosus A chronic skin condition where there is local degeneration and increased risk of tissue breakdown.

Lymphatic obstruction oedema
(SEE Lymphoedema.)

Lymphocytes Lymphocytes are the body's method of defence. They are white blood cells, produced within the lymph nodes, spleen, thymus and tonsils.

Lymphoedema A chronic swelling of the limbs due to a failure of the lymph drainage system to remove the protein rich interstitial fluid. Often occurs following surgery or radiotherapy. There is a high potential for leg ulcer development (*Figure 23*). Also known as lymphatic obstruction oedema.

Lyse To separate or split apart. In wound care streptokinase will lyse necrotic tissue.

Lysis The process of separation or splitting apart. (SEE Lyse.)

M

Maceration The softening of tissue that has remained moist or wet for a long period. The skin becomes white and soggy, (*Figure 24*) and less resilient. Can predispose to tissue breakdown. Peri-wound areas will become macerated when wound fluid or a wet dressing spills over onto good tissue and cannot dry. There is also potential for sacral tissues to be at high risk of maceration due to urine in incontinence. There is an argument for using body-worn incontinence pads with stay-dry liners to prevent maceration. Macerated tissues are in danger of excoriation and increased risk of pressure ulcer formation.

Macrophages Macrophages are phagocytic and play a role in protecting the wound against bacterial invasion. They also produce chemical mediators and are 'work-horses' as they are encouraged, in the first 24 hours, to the injured site where they lyse clots and debris, destroy and remove bacteria and allow fluid filled cavities to form, into which fibroblasts and endothelial cells can grow. Macrophages continue to play an important part in wound healing, releasing and inducing a number of polypeptide factors (cytokines) which are presently being studied in promotion of wound healing. They require a moist wound environment to enable interaction with, and migration across, the wound surface. Provision of a moist wound bed is vital for this important player to accomplish the task.

Macroscopic Visible to the naked eye.

Macrovascular Pertaining to large vessels.

Macrovascular disease Disease of the larger arteries. Usually atherosclerosis. Macrovascular disease can lead to arterial leg ulceration.

Maggot therapy Maggot (or larvae) therapy has been used for many centuries as a natural debrider of wounds and there is evidence that the benefits of maggots were noted as long ago as in 1557. (SEE Larval therapy.)

Malignancy The condition of being malignant.

Malignant In general, a disease or condition that is resistant to treatment and can often be fatal, eg. HIV AIDS, motor neurone disease, some cancers. With reference to a cancer/neoplasm, it has the capacity to invade and destroy tissues. The ability to metastasise to distant parts of the body. (SEE Malignancy and Metastasis.)

Malleoli sing. malleolus. The lateral and medial ankle bones which are sited above the foot at the base of the tibia and fibula in the leg (part of the ankle joint complex).

Malnutrition Poor nutritional status resulting from impaired absorption, poor diet or overeating. Many patients with wounds are malnourished because protein leaks away in the wound exudate. Vitamin C and zinc are a necessary part of wound healing.

Malodour Unpleasant smell, brought about by bacterial action associated with poor hygiene or wound exudate. The odour in a wound is generally an indication of the type of bacteria colonising the wound. A necrotic wound, in the process of natural debridement, will almost certainly contain anaerobic bacteria and produce a foul malodour. The malodour is due to volatile fatty acids that are the products of bacterial metabolism and, possibly putrescine and cadaverine (particularly in pressure ulcers), both of which are formed in necrotic tissue.

Malpractice Inappropriate, improper assessment and management of a patient and/or situation.

Mannuronic acid Some alginates contain mannuronic acid, which breaks down quickly in the presence of sodium and rinses away. The alginates rich in mannuronic acid form soft flexible gels. Other alginates contain guluronic acid. (SEE Guluronic acid.)

Manuka honey Produced by bees that have fed on the Manuka plant. Form of honey particularly effective in encouraging wound healing. The mode of action is thought to include release of hydrogen peroxide as well as providing sugars (glucose and fructose) to the wound site. (SEE Honey.)

Martorell's ulceration Generally occurs on the shin and is shallow with a necrotic base (*Figure 25*). Matorell ulcers are generally secondary to hypertension.

Mast cells Cells found in the tissues and filled with granules containing heparin, serotonin and histamine. These substances are released in response to inflammation or an allergic stimulation. (SEE Degranulate.) Histamine produces the redness and swelling seen immediately post injury or during an allergic episode.

Matrix (SEE Dermis and Extracellular matrix.)

Maturation phase The final stage of wound healing involves wound contraction, full epithelialisation and reorganisation.

Mechanical forces Pressure, friction and shear.

Medial On the inner side of the body.

Mediators Chemical substances that affect biological change, for example, vasoactive substances such as histamine cause vasodilation; cytokines and growth factors influence cell migration and division.

Medicated tulle dressing Contains either chlorhexidine or antibiotics. Topical antibiotics are no longer recommended in wound care due to the increased potential for bacterial sensitivity.

Medley risk assessment A method of assessing the risk of pressure ulcer formation in patients who are unwell or immobile. (SEE *Appendix*.)

Melanin Substance produced by melanocytes in the epidermis, secreted as melanosomes into keratinocytes, where they arrange supra-nuclearly as protection from ultra violet radiation. One of the substances responsible for skin colouring.

Melanoma A malignant tumour that can arise in the skin and metastasises rapidly (<6 weeks). Often has the appearance of a mole that is undergoing changes such as growth, bleeding and forming an irregular shape. Avoiding sunburn is advised to prevent these tumours.

Membrane General term for a very thin layer covering a surface, eg. of a cell.

Metabolite Product of cell respiration and metabolism, removed by the lymphatic and venous circulation.

Metalloproteinases These are peptide hydrolase enzymes which use a metal (eg. zinc) in a catalytic mechanism; they break down collagens and help to remodel extracellular matrix in healing.

Metastasis The movement of malignant disease from one part of the body (primary site) to another; movement of tumour cells may be through the lymph or blood vessels or by direct local extension. The new site of malignancy is termed 'secondary'.

Methicillin-resistant _Staphylococcus aureus_ (MRSA) _Staphylococcus aureus_ bacterium is a common infective microbe, found in about 30% of the population. It has become resistant to most antibiotics, and requires special management, mainly using vancomycin, to prevent further spread. An increasing form of MRSA is epidemic MRSA (EMRSA), (three well-defined strains of MRSA) which continues to affect hospitals in England and Wales. A new form of MRSA is vancomycin resistant (VRSA) which presents health professionals with increasing problems for management.

Metronidazole gel A hypromellose gel containing 0.8% Metronidazole (licensed for wound care), which is useful against the aerobic and anaerobic organisms that cause odour within the wound but is used mainly to combat anaerobic bacterial malodour in fungating wounds.

Microbe A micro-organism that may cause disease.

Microbiology The study of micro-organisms (bacteria, viruses and fungi) and their effect on body cells.

Microcirculation The small vessels or capillaries that deliver nutrients and oxygen to the tissue and remove unwanted waste products and fluid. It is inefficiency of the microcirculation that can lead to tissue breakdown in diabetes sufferers.

Microenvironment The immediate physical and chemical surroundings of a micro-organism.

Microfilaments Minute intercellular structures that have the appearance of threads, for example, myosin and actin.

Microflora The micro-organisms that live within the environment and body and form a necessary part of the balance. Microscopic organisms including bacteria, fungi and yeasts.

Microthrombi Microscopic blood clots that form within the smaller vessels. Microthrombi occur when sustained and unrelieved pressure is present over a bony prominence. These clots prevent blood from reaching the tissues and initiate an inflammatory response.

Microvascular Pertaining to small vessels. Microscopic vessels, often taken to refer to the capillary network.

Microvascular disease Small blood vessel disease, leading to ischaemic changes in tissues through partial occlusion of these vessels. Often found in diabetic patients (microangiopathy) or those with rheumatoid disease (vasculitis). The macrovessels of patients with leg ulcers may show a normal ABPI with Doppler ultrasound, but it could still be dangerous to use compression therapy as there could be concomitant microvascular diseases. (SEE Microcirculation.)

Migration The movement of cells from one area of a tissue or a wound to another, eg. epithelial cells during re-epithelialisation, leucocytes and macrophages during the inflammatory/extravasation phase. (SEE Epithelial tissue.)

Milton (SEE Hypochlorite).

Mitochondria Cellular units which act as the cellular 'power-house' producing energy for movement and wound healing, etc.

Mitogenic Stimulates mitosis.

Mitosis The division of cell nucleus to form daughter cells with exactly the same chromosome DNA content as that of the original cell. Mitosis in wound healing is reliant on temperature of the wound. Any drop of 2°C or more can delay mitotic activity for up to four hours.

Mitotic Relating to mitosis.

Mixed aetiology (complex aetiology) A condition that has a number of causes that may occur in any combination is said to have a mixed aetiology. The term is used to describe a wound with multiple causes, eg. a patient who has elements of both arterial and venous disease would be considered to have a wound of mixed aetiology. This would be identified through observing changes in the leg which suggest venous disease (oedema, haemosiderin, lipodermatosclerosis) and through Doppler assessment. A Doppler assessment (ABPI greater than 0.8) could indicate that certain patients receive compression therapy. An ABPI lower than 0.8 indicates arterial disease and it would be unwise to compress. (SEE Doppler.)

Modified Pütter technique A method of applying short-stretch bandages. This technique begins with two turns around the malleolus to secure the bandage then over the foot followed by one turn around the toes. The bandage is now applied at full extension and the heel and foot are covered with a figure 8 bandage. Now spiralled, at full tension, around the malleolus and one or two turns above. At the next turn, the bandage will loop around the back of the calf — approximately two fingers below the popliteal crease. Spiral down the leg beginning with a full turn at the top and then at 50% tension. If required, a second bandage can be used over the first. This would be a simple spiral technique applied in the opposite direction to the first bandage, from malleolus to two fingers below the popliteal crease.

Moist wound healing Experimental wounds have been found to heal 40% faster under an occlusive dressing than under a dry dressing. Epithelial tissue has been found to require moisture to migrate across the dermis and the tissue immediately below the occlusive dressing remained viable and moist, thereby providing the means for healing to occur. To date, scientists have been unable to quantify the optimal moisture. Moist wound healing remains the least understood term in wound care.

Moisture vapour transfer rate (MVTR) The rate at which moisture (mainly from wound exudate) passes through a dressing and evaporates into the atmosphere. The MVTR of an occlusive dressing will be little or none, whereas dry dressings will have a very high rate. The latter have no bacterial barrier and also allow the wound to dry out. Recent developments in dressing technology have produced dressings with a high MVTR that maintain a moist environment and bacterial barrier.

Mole Naevus or benign growth with increased numbers of melanocytes, has potential if irritated mechanically to become malignant.

Monocyte A white blood cell with a single nucleus. This has a phagocytic action and is responsible for cleansing the wound and protecting against infection.

Monofilament Single-strand toothbrush-type device to measure, reliably, level of peripheral sensation. A 10g monofilament is usually selected. Used to detect the degree of neuropathy (loss of sensation) in patients with diabetes and diabetic foot ulcers.

Monophasic sound When listening to a handheld Doppler to assess blood flow, only one fairly continuous sound is heard, suggestive of large vessel disease such as atherosclerosis. Can be heard during Doppler assessment when the elasticity has disappeared from an artery due to the atherosclerotic plaques that are laid down on the walls. The plaques can become very hardened and are not compressible by a sphygmomanometer. The arterial sound is highly elevated and can be double or more the systolic sound of the brachial artery. The monophasic sound heard at this time is like a dog barking, a 'woof-woof' sound.

Morphogenesis Developing, changing shape of a tissue or body site.

Motor A muscle or nerve that effects or produces movement. Lack of movement can lead to the development of pressure ulcers.

Motor neuropathy Lack of enervation to muscles. In the foot, wasting of muscles often causes *pes cavus* (cavoid foot) — a high arched foot and clawed toes. The change in shape of the foot could pre-dispose it to risk of pressure ulcer development in poorly fitting shoes.

Mould Microscopic fungi.

MRSA   (SEE   Methicillin-resistant
Staphylococcus aureus).

Multi-layer bandage Often referred to
as four-layer bandage.

Mummified Dried out — desiccated.
Dried but has maintained shape (*Figure 8*).
Preserved through drying out process. Dry
gangrene will lead to mummification of
toes or limbs. It is wise not to dress dry
gangrene with 'wet' dressings as this can
create malodour, open good tissues to
clinical   infection   and   prevent   the
mummification   process   from   natural
amputation. The patient should always be
urgently referred for vascular assessment.

Munchausen's syndrome
Inappropriate desire to seek treatment, with
clinical features, all of which are false. (SEE
Factitious wound.)

Mycosis Condition where there is topical
or systemic infection by a fungus.

Myeloperoxidase A peroxidase found
in   macrophages   and   neutrophils,
responsible   for   generating   potent
bacteriocidal activity by the hydrolysis of
hydrogen peroxide in the presence of
halide ions, such as iodine. A metallo-
enzyme containing iron. (SEE Iodine.)

Myiasis The invasion of living tissues of
man and other mammals by dipterous
larvae. (SEE Larval therapy.)

Myofibroblast A form of fibroblast
(cell involved in tissue repair) which is
motile (can move) and pulls wound tissues
together in the wound contraction phase to
reduce the volume of the wound.

Myosin A contractile protein found in
muscle.

N

NA dressings Non-adherent dressings.

Naevus Skin lesion. Spider naevus is
characterised by presence of tiny blood
vessels radiating from a central point.
Melanocytic naevus is a mole. (SEE Mole.)

Navicular Bone on the medial aspect of
the foot. In Charcot's foot, the foot
becomes mal-aligned and this bone may
take load, leading to ulceration.

Necrobiosis lipoidica A skin condition, may be seen in diabetes, where there
is degeneration of tissue, possibly leading
to tissue breakdown. Its appearance ranges
from shiny, fragile patches often on shins,
to areas of erythema and discomfort.

Necrosis Death in a tissue or an organ,
which occurs in response to injury, disease
or occlusion of blood flow. Continuity with
neighbouring viable tissue is preserved. Can
arise through infection (caseous necrosis in
tuberculosis), liquefaction from hydrolytic

enzymes, trauma such as pressure, and,
localised ischaemia. Gangrene is necrosis
associated with superinfection by putre-
fying micro-organisms. The death of tissue,
may appear blue-black, grey, yellow and
sloughy, often very painful, may have a halo
of inflammation (*Figure 26*).

Necrotic Dead tissue.

Necrotising fasciitis   A   serious
bacterial infection usually due to *Streptococcus pyogenes* but is sometimes caused
by *Staphylococcus aureus*, uncommon in
the UK, although it is more common in
Third World countries. There are a variety
of terms used to describe the infection:
hospital gangrene, suppurative fasciitis,
necrotising   erysipelas,   acute   dermal
gangrene,   Fournier's   gangrene,   acute
infective gangrene, haemolytic *Streptococcus* gangrene.

Neogenesis Regeneration of tissue.

Neoplasm New growth of tissue tumour that could be benign or malignant. Long-term non-healing leg ulcers should always be considered for biopsy, particularly if they present with cauliflower-type margins.

Neuropathic foot May occur as a complication of medical disorder, eg. diabetes or leprosy, or due to injury to the nerves. Loss of sensation means injury is not perceived, loss of motor function often results in abnormal foot position and function, loss of autonomic nerve supply affects blood supply.

Neuropathic ulcers Ulcers of the foot, most commonly associated with diabetes in the Western World. Injury is not perceived due to lack of sensation and tissue damage continues leading to tissue breakdown and overt ulceration. Neuropathic ulcers may be deep and track to other areas, often exudate is moderate to copious. In Leprosy (Hansen's disease), patients frequently present with neuropathic foot ulcers.

Neuropathy Interruption of nerve function. May result in lack of sensation, loss of motor function (eg. of muscles) or affect autonomic supply to areas such as blood vessels. Neuropathy is the commonest complication of diabetes, and usually arises within five years of the onset of the disease. Fifty per cent of patients with neuropathic joints require amputation within five years.

Neutrophils A polymorphonuclear leucocyte which has a neutral reaction to both acid and alkaline dyes. Neutrophils are white blood cells, which remove and destroy bacteria and cellular debris by the action of phagocytosis and proteolysis.

NICE National Institute of Clinical Excellence. A UK Government body with a responsibility for facilitating and monitoring clinical standards, and dissemination of related information.

Nikolsky's sign A sign noted by Polish dermatologist Pyotr Nikolsky in 1855. A clinical test, now virtually obsolete, for blistering diseases. The sign involves the production or extension of a blistering process by the combination of pressure with a sliding action, easily separating the stratum corneum layer of the epidermis from the basal layer in apparently normal skin. It is used in diagnosis of Pemphigus and Pemphigoid and some other blistering diseases, such as toxic epidermal necrolysis and epidermolysis bullosa.

Nitric oxide (NO) Substance produced by cells as part of the inflammatory and immune responses, if released inappropriately may cause tissue damage. Triggered by hypoxia. Inhibits contraction in adjacent smooth muscle. Works with prostacyclin to limit thrombus formation.

Nociceptor A nerve receptor which responds to the stimulus of injury.

Nodule Small bump (around 2cm diameter) that is palpable in the tissues.

Non-blanching erythema A reddened area of the skin, which does not turn white under finger pressure. This indicates that damage has occurred due to unrelieved pressure and that inflammatory changes are present in the tissues. The patient requires immediate intervention, such as pressure reducing equipment, increased frequency of mobilisation and repositioning schedules. Blanching hyperaemia is difficult to detect in dark or tanned skin (*Figure 27*), and physical assessment becomes important in reviewing risk in these patients, eg. heat over the area, solid or hardened tissue, darkened area of tissue.

Non-blanching hyperaemia (SEE Non-blanching erythema).

Non-compliant A subjective description of a patient who does not wish to follow treatment as prescribed. These patients are often labelled as 'non-compliant'.

Non-enzymatic glycation The mechanism by which proteins, such as collagen, form cross-linkages, associated in the presence of glucose. This makes the tissues stiffer and less able to conform to contact surfaces. This may be compensated by adjacent tissues which become over-loaded with increased risk of breakdown.

Non-ionic solution A substance which in aqueous solution has no positive or negative charge and is unlikely to be absorbed by the wound.

Non-steroidal anti-inflammatory drugs (NSAIDs) Anti-inflammatory and anal-gesic drugs based on the inhibition of cyclooxygenase pathways. This inhibits prostaglandin inflammatory mediator production. These drugs are not cortico-steroids, hence the name; examples are ibuprofen and naproxen. Used to treat osteo- and rheumatoid arthritis and other chronic inflammatory conditions, including pain associated with leg ulcers.

Normal saline A solution of 0.9% sodium chloride in sterile water; frequently used to irrigate wounds. Isotonic to the pH and molarity of tissue fluids and not absorbed by cells. Not harmful.

Normal sitting In normal sitting the pelvis is tilted slightly anteriorly, allowing the body weight to be taken through both ischial tuberosities. The hips are positioned in slight lateral rotation and flexed to an angle of 90°. The knees are also flexed to 90° and the feet are placed flat on the floor. The spine is in normal alignment with its anterior and posterior curves, and the head is positioned in the midline, facing forwards. In this position, the potential for pressure ulcer formation is reduced as weight distribution is even.

Norton risk assessment A method of assessing risk of pressure ulcer development (SEE *Appendix*). (SEE Risk assessment.)

O

Occlusion To close or to be closed, for example, a blocked blood vessel or a wound closed to the air and to moisture vapour loss, hence the term 'occlusive' dressing. Blood vessels can often become occluded by pressure, for example, when lying or sitting on a support surface. If the occlusion is not released, ie. if the person does not change his position, tissue necrosis may develop from reduced perfusion, resulting in a pressure ulcer. Occlusion can also refer to deep vein thrombosis and atherosclerosis.

Occlusive dressing An impermeable or semi-permeable wound dressing which completely covers a wound. Some examples protect the wound from the external environment, preventing microbial invasion and maintaining wound temperature. It is thought to provide a low oxygen environment which may have a positive influence on angiogenesis, as the new capillary buds grow towards a region of low oxygen tension.

Oedema An unnatural accumulation of fluid in interstitial spaces of tissue which can occur anywhere in the body. Oedema is often observed in the lower limbs of people whose deep and or superficial veins have incompetent valves. The veins become ineffective at returning blood to the heart and, as a result, venous stasis is observed in the lower leg, resulting in oedema. (SEE Lymphoedema.)

Ointments A preparation with an oily base that is applied to the external surfaces of the body. Ointments often contain drugs such as local anaesthesics or topical antimicrobials.

Onychocryptosis True in-grown nail where a spicule of nail grows into the side of the toe (nail sulcus). Infection is frequent and hypergranulation tissue can develop. Pain invariably occurs.

Onychogryphosis Thickened and deformed nail plate following sudden trauma, non-reversible, also called ram's horn nail, ostler's toe.

Optimum wound healing environment Wound healing requires a warm, moist and trauma free environment to heal. However, this state for optimum healing should not be linked to a non-healing wound, as the ideal healing environment will not promote granulation tissue unless the wound is prepared and ready to heal. To prepare the wound for healing, it must be relieved of necrotic tissue and factors that interfere with the healing process should be corrected. Once the environment is ideal, mitotic activity will commence. (SEE Ideal wound healing environment.)

Organism An individual life form such as an animal or a plant, which is able to maintain life via mutually dependent organs or organelles.

Orthopaedic wool Cotton wadding that has been formed into a bandage roll. It is used under compression bandaging or plaster of Paris in order to protect the underlying skin and bony prominences.

Osmosis The movement of fluid (eg. water) through a semipermeable membrane from an area of low solute concentration to one with a high solute concentration, until the concentration of the solutions equalise. If a wound is bathed in water, it is possible that the cells will take in water and burst.

Osmotic pressure The pressure exerted on a semi-permeable membrane by a solution.

Osteomyelitis Clinical infection sited in the bone. This often causes a sinus to form, carrying pus toward the surface tissues. Wounds that are sited close to bone can lead to osteomyelitis, eg. heel pressure ulcers, sacral pressure ulcers, dehisced knee replacement and diabetic foot ulcers.

Osteophyte Small bony outgrowth, often from a joint. Within the foot, oesteophytes may cause pressure ulcers.

Overgranulation Or proud-flesh, occurs in the later stages of healing, when the wound bed has filled with granulation tissue and normal epithelialisation does not occur. The granulation tissue continues to fill the area until it is proud of the wound, preventing epithelial tissue from migrating over the surface. Overgranulation may occur because either modern dressings are too effective at encouraging granulation tissue or a previous chronic infection has not allowed epithelialisation to 'switch on'.

Overlay A thin mattress used over the top of the patient's existing mattress. Overlays can either be static or dynamic. Static mattresses can be constructed from materials such as foam, fibre or air. Static overlays are mainly indicated for the provision of comfort and prevention of pressure ulcers in low to medium risk patients. Alternating overlays are indicated for patients who are at medium to high risk.

Overt With reference to an open lesion means superficial skin is absent and underlying tissues are exposed.

Oxford pressure monitor A device for assessing interface pressures between a bony prominence and a mattress or chair. These are often used to measure sub-bandage pressures in compression therapy.

Oxidation A biochemical process which can degrade amino acids, glucose, fatty acids, and xenobiotics such as carcinogens by enzymatic hydroxylation.

P

Paint Solution, usually containing an active ingredient, for application to the body, may be aqueous or in spirit.

Palliative care A philosophy of care that is designed to alleviate or diminish the intensity of uncomfortable symptoms.

Palpate the pulse Use of the fingers to examine the pulse to provide an indication of heart rate as well as presence of flow through the larger arteries. It is incorrect to assume that assessment of the quality of arterial flow can be achieved through palpation of the pulse. This examination should always be undertaken by Doppler assessment. However, presence of athero-sclerosis can give erroneous Doppler interpretations. (SEE Monophasic sound; ABPI.)

Palpation An examination of an area of the body using the hands. Assessment may elicit information such as temperature and texture and tissue tone/resilience.

Papilla The upward projections of the dermis into the epidermis of the skin.

Papilloma Benign overgrowth of papillae forming a tumour under the skin's surface.

Parabens A preservative contained in some creams. Can act as an allergen.

Paraffin Mineral oil. Used in paraffin and gauze dressings and white petroleum jelly and paraffin ointment mix (50–50%), etc.

Paraffin gauze Cotton or synthetic gauze impregnated with paraffin in order to prevent a dressing adhering to a wound. Paraffin gauze may easily dry out and cause adhesion, and so either several layers of the dressing should be used, or an occlusive film dressing should be used over the top. (SEE Medicated tulle dressing; Jelonet®.)

Paronychia Inflammation of the tissues surrounding the nail.

Paste Base vehicle for an active ingredient, soft but thicker than ointment or cream.

Patch test A skin test designed to characterise allergens, particularly those associated with contact dermatitis. An adhesive patch with nothing on it (serving as the control) is attached to the skin. A second patch with the potentially allergic substance placed onto it, is also attached to the skin. A positive reaction manifests as inflammation under the offending patch.

Pathogen Any micro-organism which is capable of producing disease, such as a bacterium or virus.

Pathogenesis Development of a patho-logical (abnormal) state.

Pathology The study of disease.

PDGF (SEE Platelet derived growth factors).

Pedal pulse Pertaining to the foot. The two vessels most frequently palpated are the dorsalis pedis and the posterior tibial. Used for Doppler assessment. (SEE Doppler ultrasound.)

Pelvic obliquity A common postural change associated with poor seating provision, often a saggy seat surface. The pelvis leans laterally, and much of the body weight is supported by one ischial tuberosity only, placing it at risk of pressure ulcer development. If the pelvic obliquity is severe, the body weight is also supported by the greater trochanter on the side of the obliquity, and this can result in a large pressure ulcer.

Pelvic rotation A postural change which often occurs as a result of poor seating provision, characterised by one side of the pelvis moving further forward than the other side. One ischial tuberosity is further forward than the other, and the leg on the side of the pelvis that is further forward appears longer than the other. The hip on the side of the pelvis not rotated moves forward posteriorly and laterally, off the edge of the cushion, and the trunk twists forward on the side of the pelvis that is also forward. The head follows the direction of the trunk, and the spine compensates by re-aligning itself to the front so that the head can look forwards. This results in rotation of the trunk.

Pemphigoid A similar disease to pemphigus. A distinguishing factor is that the walls of the blisters are thicker. Pemphigoid is an autoimmune disorder, effecting the dermo-epidermal junction and manifesting as large blisters that remain firm when pressed by a finger (a negative Nikolsky's sign). It is mainly a disease of the elderly, often preceded by an itchy rash, which can be mistaken for urticaria or eczema. If a blister does break, then the skin usually heals. The disease is managed with steroidal therapy, and the prognosis is usually better than pemphigus. (SEE Pemphigus.)

Pemphigus An uncommon chronic intra-epidermal blistering disease of unknown aetiology, characterised by thin walled bullae which arise from seemingly normal skin. The blisters are generally smaller than in pemphigoid and appear softer, particularly when pressed. The fluid in the blister will be seen to spread under the epidermis when firmly pressed and may even disintegrate (a positive Nikolsky's sign). Increasing numbers of blisters appear, which leave erosions once they burst. The person becomes weak and can suffer from frequent major infections and fluid loss.

Penicillin An antibiotic which targets the Gram-positive bacterial cell wall and interferes with the cell's osmotic pressure. This ensures that the cell cannot function, collapse occurs and the cell dies.

Percutaneous Performed through the skin. For example, a biopsy or insertion of fluid via a needle or catheter into the skin, or aspiration of fluid from a space below the skin.

Percutaneous absorption The method by which a topically applied substance passes through the skin.

Peri-stomal The outer margins of a stoma.

Peri-wound The outer margins of a wound.

Permeable A state of being penetrable to fluids and other substances, for example, cell membranes.

Peroneal artery An artery found in the lower limb, which originates from the popliteal artery.

Petroleum jelly Derivative of natural oil which forms an ointment base. May be impregnated into open weave gauze as a wound dressing or applied in gel form.

Phagocyte A cell with the ability to ingest bacteria, other cells and foreign particles.

Phagocytosis The method of ingestion by cells of solid material such as cellular debris, other cells, necrotic tissue and bacteria.

Phantom limb pain Pain felt in an amputated limb. The mechanism for this is poorly understood.

Pharmaceutics Relates to pharmacy and the preparation of drugs for medicinal use.

Pharmacology Study of drugs, their actions and uses.

Pharmacy Storage, preparation and dispensing of medicines.

Phases of healing There are four (or more) stages of normal wound healing: inflammation, destruction, proliferation and maturation. Although different terms may be used (eg. repair, remodelling), they all refer to the same process.

Phlebitis A painful inflammation of the vein. Can lead to thrombus formation.

Phonophoresis Use of ultrasound to enhance percutaneous absorption (to drive) of topically applied substances through the skin. Also called iontophoresis.

Photoplethysmography A method of using doppler to monitor blood flow changes. (SEE Venous occlusion plethysmography.)

Pigmentation A colouration of the skin which occurs naturally, for example, melanin.

Pilonidal sinus Usually found on the coccyx. Caused by a hair that folds back on itself and grows into the tissue and becomes infected. Often treated by surgery.

Pinch grafting Small pinches of skin can be harvested by the use of a scalpel and forceps and then sited in patches onto an ulcer. Pinch grafting is simple and can be achieved easily at the bedside or in the home. Local anaesthetic is injected prior to harvesting.

Pink wound The stage of healing or non-healing is sometimes identified through wound colour. This is a subjective method and is not accurate but can be helpful in noting wound changes during assessment and documentation. A pink wound is one that is in the final stages of healing and contains epithelial tissue (*Figure 28*). (SEE Red wound, Yellow wound, Green wound, Black wound.)

Plantar warts Also known as verrucae, infection by human papilloma virus causes hyperplasia of epidermal cells creating a benign tumour.

Plasmid A small, independently replicating, piece of extrachromosomal DNA that can be transferred from one organism to another. Plasmids carrying antibiotic resistant genes can spread this trait rapidly through the population. Described largely from bacteria and protozoa. Some plasmids are capable of integrating into the host genome.

Plasminogen activators Plasminogen is the pro-enzyme of plasmin and promotes fibrinolysis and cell migration during normal wound healing.

Plasminogen activator inhibitor Initiates a proteolytic cascade, resulting in activation of matrix metalloproteinases *in vitro*, leading to degradation of extra-cellular matrix.

Plastic surgery Surgery aimed at restoring, altering or replacing visible areas of the body. In wound care, plastic surgery may involve the use of skin grafts in order to close wounds more effectively than if left to heal naturally.

Platelet derived growth factors (PDGF) Is released into a wound by degranulating platelets and is a mitogen and chemotaxin for fibroblasts.

Platelets Found in the blood, contain granules which are released following injury to initiate the clotting cascade. Platelets do not contain a nucleus. Are responsible for PDGF. (SEE Platelet derived growth factors.)

Plaques An area of atherosclerosis. Or, a flat and often raised patch on the skin or any other organ of the body.

Plexus A 'braid'. A term describing an organisation produced by the intertwining of blood vessels or nerves. Network, used in relation to capillary network.

Pneumatic intermittent compression A method of compression therapy applied in the form of an inflatable boot, which provides sequential intermittent compression. It is used as an addition to other treatment regimes in reducing limb oedema, and may be applied once or twice per day.

Polymer Repeated chains of molecules to form a substance, eg. polyethylene (polythene) is a polymer.

Polymorphonucleocytes White blood cells with deeply lobed nuclei.

Polypeptide factors (SEE Cytokines or growth factors).

Polysaccharide beads Wound care product poured into the wound cavity to absorb exudate.

Polyurethane foam A type of foam which can be open cell or closed cell in its construction. It is used in the manufacture of pressure-reducing mattresses and cushions, and also wound dressings.

Popliteal artery An artery found in the lower limb which originates from the femoral artery.

Popliteal fossa The hollow area on the posterior aspect of the knee joint when the knee is flexed, such as in sitting. It contains both the tibial nerve and popliteal artery, which can become easily compressed if seat depth is too long, leading to increased potential for DVT.

Positive Stemmer's sign If the lymphatic system is unable to perform its function, oedema is the result. The oedema is hard to the touch and does not 'pit' when pressed and the skin between the toes cannot be pinched.

Posterior pelvic tilt Probably the most common postural change associated with sitting for long periods of time. Sitting in a posterior pelvic tilt will reduce functional ability, and increase risk of pressure ulcer development due to the excessive loading of areas of the body that cannot withstand this. There are three major causes of posterior pelvic tilt.

1. Sitting for long periods of time will succumb to the effects of gravity and slide down in the chair.
2. The armchair or wheelchair could cause the posture to develop.
3. The person's physical condition may result in a tendency to adopt a posterior pelvic tilt.

In a posterior pelvic tilt the pelvis rotates posteriorly, and so the sacrum and coccyx support a large percentage of body weight. The hip angle opens, moving the thighs forwards off the chair. The angle at the knees and ankle also increases, and the feet can no longer be easily placed flat on the floor. They push forwards, supporting much of the weight of the lower limbs on the heels, thereby placing them at an increased risk of pressure ulcers. The head realigns itself forwards over the pelvis, causing the spine to compensate, becoming rounded in shape, and a kyphosis will develop. The internal organs therefore become compressed.

Posterior superior iliac spines (PSISs) These processes are found on the posterior aspect of the pelvis, either side of the sacrum. In a neutral sitting position the PSISs sit at the same height as the anterior superior iliac spines (ASISs) when viewed/palpated from a lateral position, and provide useful information on the position of the pelvis during a seating assessment.

Posterior tibial artery A branch of the popliteal artery, found in the lower limb.

Posture Posture is usually defined as the positions of trunk, head and the limbs in relation to each other. 'Normal' posture varies from person to person, and is dependent on muscle capabilities, a sense of awareness of where the body is in space, and the ability to maintain balance. Individuals adopt many different postures during the day depending on the tasks being performed by them at any one time. Due to muscle fatigue, no single posture can be maintained for long periods of time.

Postural change A change to normal skeletal alignment, often due to poor sitting position (but also due to other causes such as increased muscle tone). Postural changes may be flexible and, as such, correctable with the use of seating systems, or fixed postural changes. Fixed postural changes are permanent and cannot be corrected. They must therefore be accommodated.

Potassium permanganate (KMnO$_4$) A dark purple water-soluble compound which is used as a disinfectant and deodorant and for cleaning wounds. It is thought to be indicated in assisting the dehydration of very wet wounds and eczema, but there is little clinical evidence to support this theory.

Prednisolone Systemic steroid therapy used in the treatment of rheumatoid arthritis and asthma. Long-term steroid therapy will reduce the production of prostaglandins. Prostaglandins have a role in wound healing and the interference of steroids in this process can delay wound healing. Long-term therapy will also cause the skin to be paper thin and easily traumatised.

Pressure Also referred to as interface pressure. Pressure ulcers develop as a result of occlusion of blood vessels by external pressure, and endothelial damage of arterioles and the microcirculation due to the application of friction and shearing forces. Pressure is calculated using the following formula: pressure equals force divided by the surface area. Pressure compresses the skin and internal tissues between the bone and the support surface, causing ischaemia, which, if continued, will result in cell death. Landis (1931) described the average level of pressure required to close the capillaries as between 16– 32mmHg. In a healthy person, once pressure has occluded the capillaries, the tissues become starved of oxygen and nutrients. Pain signals are sent to the brain, which in turn consciously or unconsciously informs the person to change position. As soon as the position is changed, blood supply is restored to the occluded area, preventing skin damage and restoring comfort. In those people whose health is compromised, this continual repositioning can be painful and distressing. There is some evidence to suggest that interface pressures are three to five times greater at the bone than at the skin surface. This creates a 'cone of pressure' (SEE Cone of pressure), and causes tissue damage at the bone before it is noted at the skin surface. At this interface some slipping or sliding (shear forces and friction) may also be present, which can increase tissue damage. Manufacturers provide information about interface pressure measurements related to their mattresses. However, this is not a safe method of judging mattresses as interface pressures are not clinically relevant.

Pressure distribution In order for interface pressure to be minimised, the body surface needs to be supported as much as possible, distributing the pressure over a greater surface area of the body. Pressure distribution is good in a recumbent position, as a large percentage of the body surface area is being supported. Pressure distribution in the seated person is limited due to the small surface area in contact with the seat surface, ie. the buttocks and thighs.

Pressure necrosis Tissue death caused by unrelieved pressure.

Pressure reducing Type of equipment used in pressure ulcer prevention which aims to reduce interface pressure by supporting as much of the body surface area as possible. This equipment is also known as static equipment.

Pressure reduction Reduction of interface pressures achieved through the use of pressure reducing equipment. It is the redistribution of pressure that reduces the amount of pressure found on bony prominences. An analogy would be a diver who experiences extreme high-pressures when under water but never develops pressure ulcers because the high pressure is uniformly spread over the surface of his body. A foam or air surface provides a 'flow' similar to the water and spreads the pressure load.

Pressure relief Removal of the source of interface pressure, normally achieved through repositioning of the body surface. For example, moving from sitting to standing, or a wheelchair user who is able to carry out 'lift offs' by lifting his pelvis off the seat surface for a short period of time. As pressure is removed from the support surface, blood flow is restored to the tissues, maintaining their integrity.

Pressure relieving Pertaining to equipment which provides pressure relief, ie. alternating mattresses and cushions. These operate by inflation and deflation of individual cells, giving pressure relief over the fully deflated cell.

Prevalence An epidemiological term describing the proportion of a defined group in the population having a condition at one point in time. It is an appropriate measure only in relatively stable conditions, for example, chronic bronchitis — and is not suitable for measuring chronic wounds.

Primary dressing A dressing that is placed in immediate contact with the wound bed.

Primary intention Also known as first intention healing. A wound with edges that have been sharply incised (ie. scalpel) and has the edges brought together in approximation will heal through primary intention. Within 24 to 48 hours, the epidermis would have sealed the surface and healing will continue below this surface. When the wound is sealed by primary intention, baths and showers are possible after the 24 to 48-hour period.

Proflavin A wound cleansing product in the form of aqueous cream or a lotion, which has a mild bacteristatic effect on Gram-positive organisms, but not on Gram-negative bacteria. Limited clinical evidence is available to demonstrate its efficacy. Proflavine has no effect on the wound bacteria, as the bacteriostatic is not released into the wound bed. There is now evidence that proflavin is mutagenic, raising concerns about its safety. There is also evidence that the continued use of proflavin gauze as a wound packing is no longer justifiable.

Prognosis The expected/inevitable outcome of a condition.

Proliferation The rapid multiplication or reproduction of similar cells.

Proliferative phase The third phase of wound healing. This stage lasts three to 24 days and, during this time, there is an intense proliferation of fibroblasts and endothelial cells. Proliferating fibroblasts synthesise collagen and a collagen matrix is laid down. Endothelial buds grow into the space cleared by macrophages and the fibroblasts carry on the process of repair by laying down fibrous tissue. However, fibroblasts must be stimulated to synthesise collagen and the primary stimulants are ascorbate (ascorbic acid) and lactate, leading to many practitioners recommending vitamin C for all patients with a wound. A wound that is in healing phase 3 will possibly have a pink wound bed with dark red raised bumps in the surface with the appearance of granules, known as granulation tissue.

Prominence (SEE Bony prominence).

Prone Lying face down.

Pronation In the foot, this is an in-rolled position and the foot looks flat. Pronation is a normal part of stance phase in gait (walking), over-pronation can cause pain and overloading of some parts of the foot increasing the potential for ulceration.

Prophylaxis Protection against disease. Prophylaxis against wound infection can be achieved by preventing the access of pathogens to the body, eg. by chemical or barrier means.

Propolis Is a bee product. High in flavanoids. It is a powerful natural antibiotic, specifically against *Staphylococcus aureus*. It acts as an antioxidant free-radical scavenger.

Prostacyclin An unstable prostaglandin released by mast cells and endothelium, a potent inhibitor of platelet aggregation, also causes vasodilation and increased vascular permeability.

Prostaglandins Prostaglandins are synthesised from phospholipid fatty acids in the cell membrane through enzymic action and are promoters of the inflammatory process (drugs, such as aspirin and NSAIDs, that interfere with the production of prostaglandins will reduce inflammation). Prostaglandins act:

❖ as vasoconstrictors or vasodilators

❖ as initiators of the clotting cascade by causing platelet aggravation

❖ to influence cell activity by acting as messengers between cells

❖ to modulate intracellular activity

❖ as initiators of pain.

As prostaglandins are promoters of the inflammatory process and influence cell activity by acting as messengers between cells, any reduction in their production can have an adverse effect on healing.

Prosthesis An artificial replacement for a part of a body that is missing, such as a limb.

Protease An enzyme that breaks down proteins.

Proteins Large molecules, which consist of long sequences of amino acids, linked together by peptide bonds. Dietary protein is used for the growth and repair of body cells and tissues; synthesis of enzymes, antibodies, some hormones and plasma proteins; and less importantly, the provision of energy. Patients with long-standing large wounds may require dietary protein supplement to replace that lost in exudate, for example.

Proteolysis A process by which the protein molecule is broken down by water being added to the peptide bonds.

Proteolytic enzymes Enzymes that promote the breakdown of protein. Some proteolytic enzymes are involved in the remodelling phase of wound healing, eg. matrix metalloproteinases.

Proximal Nearer to the point of origin or the trunk. For example, the elbow is proximal to the fingers.

Pruritus Itching.

Pseudomonas aeruginosa A Gram-negative bacterium — a motile rod that will rapidly colonise humidifiers, sinks and buckets of water. Wounds colonised by this organism are likely to have (sometimes almost fluorescent) green exudate and the wound will be malodorous with a musty, distinctive and almost sweet odour.

Pseudomonas aeruginosa responds to the application of silver dressings. (SEE Silver.)

Pump (calf muscle and foot) The calf muscle pump involves the muscles of the lower leg which, in contraction, provide intermittent compression of the deep veins. This encourages blood movement back to the heart. A similar pumping mechanism occurs in the sole of the foot with compression and release during gait. Thus, movement is a helpful part of managing chronic ulceration in that it encourages venous drainage, but this must be coupled with a good understanding of other factors when taken into account in managing a chronic wound.

Pus A product of inflammation, most frequently caused by infection. It contains an abundance of used polymorphonuclear leucocytes, tissue elements liquefied by enzymes and cellular debris. The nature of the pus varies with prevalent pathogens, eg. *Staphylococcus aureus* forms a thick yellow-white pus, haemolytic *streptococcus* exudate is often thin and straw coloured.

Pyoderma gangrenosum A rare, destructive, inflammatory ulcer, probably fundamentally an autoimmunological problem, particularly as it is often found in patients with rheumatoid arthritis or inflammatory bowel disease. The clinical appearance is unique. It generally has smooth symmetrical outlines with a border of blue directly around the margins of the wound. The wound bed can often contain slough and necrotic tissue that remains hydrated. The wounds can appear anywhere on the body but are most commonly found on the proximal part of the calf.

Pyrexia A fever — the body temperature rises above normal due to disease or infection. With infection the rise in temperature can have a positive effect, as multiplication of bacteria is inhibited if body temperature is too warm. Metabolic activity is increased by 7% for each degree of celsius above the normal range.

Q

Quality adjusted life year (QALY)

A QALY is a year of life adjusted for its quality or its value. A year in perfect health is considered equal to 1.0 qaly. The value of a year in ill health would be discounted. For example, a year bedridden might have a value equal to 0.5 qaly.

Quality of life

Refers to the level of comfort, enjoyment, ability to pursue daily activities. Often used in discussions of treatment options and used as a measure of effectiveness of an intervention in clinical trials on wound care.

Quorum sensing

Is the term given to the phenomenon of microbial communication. Organisms can sense when a certain population density has developed and can prepare for a change in their environment. In the context of wound infection, this may relate to the virulence of different species at given population densities yet to be defined.

R

Randomised controlled trial

The so-called 'gold standard' of clinical evidence. This is a comparison of two or more interventions involving a random allocation of consenting patients to treatment to avoid bias. Such studies must be rigorously conducted with detailed statistical input in order to maximise the opportunity to draw meaningful conclusions from the outcome. Very few aspects of wound care are currently supported by data from RCTs.

RCT

(SEE Randomised controlled trial).

Reactive hyperaemia

Observed as a red flushing of the tissues following a period of occlusion and ischaemia. The flushing visible on the skin is the body's method of overcompensating for blood deficiency in the tissues. This ensures that the insulted tissues are provided with increased O_2, and nutrients and wounds will be supplied with the ingredients of healing. Occurs as a result of microcirculatory disruption and inflammation.

Recalcitrant wound

Unresponsive to treatment. A wound which is reluctant and difficult to heal.

Receptors

Structures on the cell surface which receive specific chemicals supplied by the blood, or:

- a sensory nerve ending
- a particular cellular protein that must bind to a hormone before a cellular response can be obtained
- a chemical structure on a cell surface, which can combine with an antigen in order to produce a distinct immunological component.

Red wound

The stage of healing or non-healing is sometimes identified through wound colour. This is a subjective method and is not accurate but can be helpful in noting wound changes during assessment and documentation. A red wound (*Figure 29*) is generally a healing (granulating) wound and requires protection. (SEE Black wound, Yellow wound, Green wound, Pink wound.)

Re-epithelialisation Re-development of new epithelial tissue following wound healing. Re-growth of the epidermis across a wound bed.

Reperfusion The restoration of passage of fluid through an organ or vessel following occlusion. For example, restoration of blood flow once interface pressure is removed.

Resect Surgical removal of a significant part of an organ or tissue.

Resistance 1. Micro-organisms, such as bacteria and viruses can develop resistance to antimicrobial/antibiotic drugs through the evolutionary process of natural selection. Injudicious use of antibiotics can select for resistance, as has occurred with methicillin in MRSA. 2. The resistance to force, such as the resistance offered by the peripheral vessels to the blood flow of the larger vessels in the circulatory system.

Resolve The abnormal condition returns to normal.

Rete peg Downward projection of the epidermis into the dermis.

Retrocalcaneal Behind the calcaneus (heel bone), just below the tendoachilles insertion.

Revascularisation The re-growth of new blood vessels within a tissue.

Rheology Study of flow of materials, eg. of blood. Blood is a thixotrophic substance and requires pressure to get it moving, the slower the flow, the more effort is required to keep it moving along the vessels.

Rheumatoid arthritis An autoimmune disorder affecting the joints, causing pain, deformity and disability. Delays healing because the disease also affects the micro-circulation within the tissues, lowering the supply of nutrients and O_2 to the wound bed.

RICE Rest Ice Compression Elevation, the recommended management for an acute inflammatory condition such as a sprained ankle.

Ringer's solution An isotonic solution that contains Ca^{2+}, K^+, Na^+, Cl^- ions. It is sometimes used to re-establish electrolyte balance. Because it is an isotonic solution, it may be preferable to using tap water for cleansing wounds.

Rodent ulcer (SEE Basal cell carcinoma).

Rubor Latin term for redness, as seen in inflammation.

Rule of nines The extent of a burned area is described by a percentage that indicates the amount of surface area involved: head, 9%; front, 18%; back, 18%; arms, 9% each; legs, 9% each; pubic area, 1%.

S

Sacro-iliac joint A planar joint which attaches the pelvic girdle to the spinal column.

Sacrum The lowest portion of the spinal column, often a location of pressure ulceration.

Salicylic acid May be used in 'corn plasters'. To be avoided in the 'at risk foot' because of its keratolytic action on skin,

which may lead to tissue damage and ulceration.

Salt Sodium chloride (NaCl), cooking salt.

Scab Dried serous exudate following injury to the skin which has caused bleeding. Re-epithelialisation occurs under the scab, which lifts off in time. As the scab evaporates, it draws fluid from the wound bed and this also evaporates. As wounds heal faster in a moist environment, it is considered wise to prevent scab formation through application of a moist dressing. (SEE Eschar.)

Scald A superficial burn wound caused by hot liquid or steam.

Scale 1. In dermatology, a flake arising from the stratum corneum. 2. A research or clinical measurement tool, eg. visual analogue scale for pain measurement.

Scar Final stage of wound healing. (SEE Hypertrophic scar and Keloid scar.)

Sclerosis A condition where the tissues harden.

Scoliosis A lateral curvature of the spine caused either by a congenital abnormality, or as a compensatory measure, for example, from sitting with a pelvic obliquity.

Screening A method of assessing the population in a routine manner.

Seat depth The correct seat depth is ascertained by measuring from the back of the buttocks to one inch behind the back of the knee. This allows the thigh to be fully supported. A seat depth which is too great will cause the patient to slide downwards in the chair in order to escape the discomfort felt at the back of the knee. As a consequence, the patient adopts a posterior pelvic tilt, risking pressure ulcer development. An insufficient seat depth provides inadequate support to the thigh and increases interface pressures on the buttocks, causing great discomfort.

Seat height The seat to ground height of a chair is calculated by measuring the length of the patient's lower leg from knee to floor. It is important that normal footwear is worn during the assessment. A seat that is too high will result in the feet being unsupported. This increases interface pressures on the buttocks and thighs, and reduces sitting stability. The patient adopts a posterior pelvic tilt as he attempts to reach the floor with his feet. A seat which is too low will result in the thighs being unsupported by the chair, and will increase interface pressures under the buttocks.

Seat width An optimum seat width allows for approximately 3cm clearance either side of the widest points of the patient's thighs, usually the trochanters. A seat that is too narrow will prevent the patient from transferring, either independently or by use of a hoist. It may also increase pressure over the greater trochanter. A seat width which is too wide will often prompt the person to fill the whole chair, by leaning to one side in order to increase sitting stability. This causes them to adopt a pelvic obliquity.

Secondary dressing A dressing used over the top of one that is already in contact with the wound bed. Often used to secure a primary dressing, to provide occlusion of the wound, or to provide additional absorptive capacity.

Secondary intention Wounds that are open either because tissue has been lost or because sides cannot be brought into close apposition for suturing may heal by secondary intention. Examples are chronic wounds and surgical incision wounds that have dehisced.

Sensitivity 1. Test for bacterial responsiveness to an antibiotic. 2. Sensitivity of a test is the precision/accuracy of a test. An accurate risk assessment scoring system will correctly identify the patients who go on to develop ulcers; or, 3. can mean cutaneous reaction to ingredients, creams or dressings (also usually known as hypersensitivity).

Sensory neuropathy Damage to the sensory nerves in the legs and feet, leading to loss of sensation and potential injury, which remains unnoticed. Frequently associated with diabetes.

Sepsis A presence of pathogenic organisms in the blood or tissues.

Septicaemia Presence of pathogenic organisms or toxins in the bloodstream.

Sequestrum pl. sequestrae. For example, bony sequestrum where a dead portion of bone has split off. Unless removed this will delay healing and may become a focus of infection.

Serotonin or 5-hydroxytryptamine (5-HT) A neurotransmitter and hormone which has vasoconstrictor properties (released from damaged platelets).

Serum albumin The serum level of the low molecular weight protein albumin. Albumin, produced by the liver, plays an important role in maintaining plasma osmotic pressure. Normal serum albumin should be 3.5–5.0 grams per decilitre. Low serum albumin can be found in cases of liver disease and malnutrition and is associated with impaired wound healing.

Sharp debridement A method of debridement, using a scalpel or scissors to separate necrotic tissue from a wound bed (*Figure 30*).

Shear forces Are uniaxial forces which act on the body from one direction only and cause tissue deformation. This may lead to damage, for example, to small blood vessels. Shear forces are most dangerous in the bedridden patient who is semi-recumbent and in the seated individual, as they have an increased risk of sliding downwards in the bed or seat. Gravity pushes down on the body encouraging it to slump and slide down in the chair or bed. While the skin remains still at the seat surface, the skeleton begins to slide down within the tissues. If interface pressures are also present, the bony prominences of the skeleton, for example, the ischial tuberosities and sacrum, rub and distort the internal tissues, causing damage. This distortion causes the capillaries to break and, as a consequence, the tissues are denied oxygen and nutrients; tissue death ensues. There may be little sign of this damage at the skin surface initially, other than a small red mark, and often, a deep pressure ulcer is revealed when the skin breaks down.

Shear stress (SEE Shear forces).

Sheepskin A product used to provide comfort in the bed or chair. Often used as a soft layer to minimise the effects of prolonged compression. There is little clinical evidence to support its use as a pressure-reducing product.

Shock-absorption A material is used to absorb the effects of sudden loading.

Short-stretch bandages A method of compression bandaging designed to promote increased venous return, allowing the tissues of the lower extremity to recover from venous hypertension. Short-stretch bandages are made from non-allergenic cotton, with the weave of the bandage giving it its extensibility. The weave of the bandage ensures that the material will only stretch a short way, hence the name, 'short-stretch'. Short-stretch bandages are applied at full stretch, and provide a rigid circumferential constraint around the leg. When the muscle contracts, it works against this constraint and rebounds. The rebound action causes the muscle to massage the deep vein thereby returning the blood to the heart. Short-stretch bandaging offers similar healing rates to multi-layer bandaging.

Sickle cell anaemia A form of anaemia so-called because of the sickle shape of the red blood cells. It is caused by the presence of an abnormal haemoglobin. Symptoms include ulceration of the lower extremities.

Silicone Any of a group of polymers made of oxygen and silicon in plastic form. Silicone is the basis of some non-adherent dressings.

Silver (Ag) Man has been aware of the medicinal and preservative properties of silver for thousands of years. The ancient Greek and Roman civilisations used silver vessels to keep drinking water potable. Silver has been used as a bactericidal since the late nineteenth century when silver nitrate drops were used for the treatment of gonorrhoeal opthalmia in newborn children. The chemical forms used have been inorganic salts, such as silver nitrate, as well as elemental and colloidal silver. Silver, in the sulphadiazine compound (SEE Silver sulphadiazine), is incorporated into creams and ointments and, in the metallic form, into a number of wound dressings. Silver has been found to be effective against a wide range of bacterial, fungal and even viral pathogens. It is generally recognised as a broad-spectrum agent with no reports of resistance and few clinical side-effects; only irritation and skin discolouration reported for the nitrate solution. The nitrate, in solution, has been used to reduce overgranulation, however, this practice has now been superceded. Silver acts biochemically as a heavy metal by impairing the bacterial electron transport system and some of its DNA functions. To do this, the 'active' agents — the silver ions — have to be bioavailable (ie. able to enter the cell) at the correct concentration in solution. In the cell membrane and cytoplasm, silver ions affect critical functional and structural proteins located both in the cell membrane and the cytoplasm. This reduces the ability of the micro-organism to maintain its cell integrity, resulting in leakage of constituents and eventual cell death.

Silver nitrate A caustic used for the reduction of hypergranulation and removal of warts. Due to the caustic nature, it is not often used for hypergranulation although it remains one of the fastest reduction methods (apart from surgery).

Silver sulphadiazine The chemical esterification of antimicrobial silver with a sulphonamide bacteriostatic agent — sulphadiazine — has resulted in a very safe broad-spectrum agent for topical use. Silver is released slowly from the oil-in-water cream formulations in concentrations that are selectively toxic to micro-organisms, such as bacteria. One per cent silver sulphadiazine cream is used for its broad-spectrum antibacterial effect and is particularly effective against Gram-negative organisms such as *Pseudomonas aeruginosa*. It has become a mainstay in the treatment of burns and has been used successfully in the treatment of leg ulcers. The cream is applied to the wound using a sterile spatula or may be spread directly onto a large dressing and placed over the wound area. The cream needs to be reapplied every 24–48 hours in order to achieve its therapeutic effect.

Sinus An epithelial cell-lined tube from the outside of the body to inside, sometimes to specific structures such as a bursa. A track to the body surface from an abscess used for the escape of pus, or an irritant material (such as suture material) which becomes the focus for an infection.

Skin The skin is the largest organ in the body, weighing 2.7kgs in the average adult, is vital to the maintenance and balance of the body and is an indispensable structure for human life. The skin has a stratified, impermeable and avascular layer, epidermis, which is waterproof, prevents water loss and acts as a barrier against bacterial invasion of dermis.

Skin flora Micro-organisms that inhabit the epidermis of the skin. A number of microbes are normally present on the skin's surface. If not pathogenic, these are known as commensals.

Skin graft Skin that is harvested from one part of the body to cover a defect in another. Used to cover burns and to promote healing in recalcitrant wounds. Skin grafts lose collagen at the same rate, regardless of thickness. Thin full-thickness grafts perform better than thick full-thickness grafts or split-thickness grafts. Meshing the graft assists with 'take'.

Skin glue Cyanoacrylate adhesive used to secure clean traumatic wounds, eg. Dermabond®.

Skin integrity The healthy skin is intact and robust. It is important to maintain healthy skin tissue; for example, by the provision of pressure reducing equipment and good exudate management to avoid maceration.

Sleek A pink adhesive plastic tape. Little used in modern wound care as the adherence can cause skin trauma. Used to attach a special nylon sheet/bag over hydro-colloid wafer when larval therapy is being used, in order to prevent the larvae from leaving the wound site.

Slough A mixture of dead white cells, dead bacteria, rehydrated necrotic tissue and fibrous tissue. Can be 'soft' slough and easily cleaned away, or fibrous slough which can resist even sharp debridement (*Figure 30*).

Slow recovery foam (SEE Visco-elastic foam).

Smoking Lowers the temperature of the skin and any drop of temperature in the wound will delay healing for up to four hours. Smoking also causes vasoconstriction and a reduction in fibrolynitic activity with an increase in the viscosity of the blood. Carbon monoxide binds to haemoglobin with an affinity 200 times that of oxygen and this lowers available oxygen to be utilised by the tissues. There can be no doubt that the reduction of nutrients and oxygen delays wound healing severely and increases the potential for clinical infection.

Solar actinosis Skin damage from prolonged exposure to ultraviolet light, shows as thickening and wrinkling, similar to solar keratosis.

Sorbitol pathways Occurs in altered glucose metabolism as in diabetes.

Sore General name for a skin abnormality or lesion.

Specificity A test that identifies those patients considered to be 'not at risk' and qualifies how many of these go on to produce a pressure ulcer. An accurate risk assessment scoring system will correctly identify those who will not develop a pressure ulcer.

Sphygmomanometer An instrument used to measure blood pressure.

Spider naevus A permanent dilation of superficial groups of capillaries or venules. They are characterised by small blood vessels radiating from a central tiny red dot. (SEE Ankle flare and naevus.)

Spinal alignment The anatomical alignment of the spine, with its anterior and posterior curves.

Squamous Usually refers in this context to flat cells, viz squamous epithelium (skin).

Staphylococcus aureus A common infecting micro-organism (pathogen) and a regular coloniser of wounds. A non-motile Gram-positive bacteria, spherical in shape and clustered together like bunches of grapes. It is found in 30–50% of the population, normally in the nasal passage, the groin or the axilla. It is an opportunistic pathogen, which destroys tissues by forming an abscess. (SEE MRSA.)

Starling's law The capillaries reabsorb 90% of the fluid released by the arteries. Blood albumin has a large part to play in this re-absorption as it creates a negative pressure within the capillary. Low serum blood albumin leads to oedema.

Stasis No flow, stopped, standing still.

Static air mattress An air-filled mattress that does not alternate intermittently.

Steroid therapy Systemic and topical steroid therapy lowers the production of prostaglandins and can produce paper-thin skin (atrophy), causing the skin to be easily damaged with degloving injuries being a common occurrence and tissues that are difficult to heal.

Stockinet A fine gauze tubular bandage. A tubular secondary dressing.

Stoma Any natural opening in the skin surface (ie. mouth, anus) or an artificially formed opening such as a colostomy, ileostomy, urostomy or tracheostomy.

Streptococcus pl. *streptococci*. A Gram-positive bacterium, oval in shape and unites together like strings of beads. Some *streptococci* discolour or destroy red blood cells and are haemolytic *streptococci*. A wound infected by haemolytic *streptococci* is likely to be beefy or brick red in colour and possibly painful and friable. It is the second most common bacterium found in wounds.

Streptodornase Is a proteolytic enzyme that liquefies the viscous nucleoprotein of dead cells or pus.

Streptokinase A thrombolytic enzyme which acts directly on a substrate of fibrin by activating a fibrinolytic enzyme in human serum breaking up thrombi.

Stress Physiological and psychological stress cause vasoconstriction, and the lowered blood delivery can affect the required nutrient supply to the wound bed.

Strike through Evidence of wound exudate appearing on the outer surface of the wound dressing, indicating a need for dressing change. Or, evidence of fluids entering through a mattress cover and contaminating the foam. Strike through in a wound dressing is believed to be associated with wound infection. Exudate saturating a non-occlusive dressing which does not have a bacterial barrier is believed to act as a portal for the ingress of pathogens.

Sub-bandage pressure The amount of pressure achieved through the bandaging process. Recommended sub-bandage pressures for venous ulcer treatment are 40mmHg at the ankle, decreasing gradually to 17mmHg at the knee. These pressures are achieved through applying the bandage under consistent tension. (SEE Laplace's law.)

Subcutaneous Beneath the epidermal and dermal layers of the skin.

Sugar paste A mixture of sugar and water with additions of either hydrogen peroxide or iodine. Sugar exerts a lethal osmotic effect on bacteria and destroys the internal cell water thereby killing the bacteria. Used on heavily exuding and malodorous wounds in order to cleanse the wound and reduce levels of exudate. Requires a secondary dressing. Can be painful, patients often experience a 'drawing' sensation.

Superficial burn The skin is dry, intact but reddened and painful. Blanches when pressed and may blister within 48 hours.

Superficial-partial thickness burn Blisters immediately and can be moist and very painful. Will be reddened but may still blanch when pressed.

Supine Lying face up.

Surgical wound Created through surgery, usually refers to a wound created by a scalpel which will heal by first intention healing. (SEE Primary intention.)

Surgical debridement Slough or necrotic tissue removed surgically either under general or local anaesthesia. (SEE Sharp debridement.)

Sustained pressure Weight or load is applied continuously. Prolonged interface pressures, such as those experienced when lying or sitting in one position for a prolonged period of time. Sustained pressure can result in tissue necrosis and is considered one of the highest risk factors in pressure ulcer formation.

Swab 1. Gauze pad that has traditionally been used to clean a wound, although no longer advised, as cotton gauze sheds fibres into the wound and the mechanical action of cleansing the wound can lead to tissue trauma and delayed healing. 2. A method of obtaining microbiological data from the wound. Is unlikely to provide reliable, quantitative or qualitative information on bacteria in a clinically infected wound as the bacteria is sited within the tissues. All chronic wounds are colonised and a swab will disclose the colonising bacteria qualitatively and semi-quantitatively. In general, antibiotics are not required for a colonised wound, they should be reserved for the treatment of spreading cellulitis.

Systemic Referring to the whole of the body rather than one component.

T

Talipes equinovarus Congenital deformity of 'club-foot'.

Talus Bone which fits beneath the tibia and fibula to form part of the ankle joint complex.

Talley monitor A device for assessing interface pressures between a bony prominence and a mattress or chair.

Tap water Tap water is used to cleanse the legs of patients with leg ulcers. Buckets are lined with polythene bags and filled with tap water. The legs should be soaked for less than five minutes as osmosis can cause cells to swell and burst. There is no evidence to suggest that tap water causes clinical infections.

Tea tree oil A topical herbal preparation which appears to have some antimicrobial action. This claim needs further confirming research. The oil, when applied topically to the skin, has sensitisation potential.

Tekscan A device for assessing and measuring interface pressures between a bony prominence and a mattress or chair. The device provides information in the form of a map showing areas of high pressure.

Telangectasia Cluster of small, thread-like veins.

Telemedicine Video link from the patient to a distant 'expert' for diagnosis, surgery, etc.

Tendonitis Inflammation of the tendon.

Tenosynovitis Inflammation of the tendon sheath.

Tensile Capable of being stretched without tearing. Refers to tissues under tension. (SEE Tensile strength.)

Tensile strength The amount of pressure that can be applied without breaking the tissues. It can refer to post healing and relates to the strength within the wound.

Tension stress Where one side of the skin site is pulled away from the other.

Thermography Non-invasive method of observing skin temperature changes.

Thermo-reactive foam (SEE Visco-elastic foam).

Thermoreceptors A heat sensitive receptor. Feedback from thermoreceptors contribute to the maintenance of body temperature.

Thirty-degree tilt Pressure ulcers primarily form over bony prominences. The 30-degree tilt places the patient at a slight angle with the use of pillows. This position places the patient onto fleshy parts of the body (ie. gluteus maximus) and removes them from bony prominences.

Thoracic support (SEE Lateral support).

Thrombocytopenia A decrease in the number of platelets in the blood, resulting in the potential for increased bleeding and decreased ability for clotting. Associated with impaired healing.

Thrombolytic Substance which has the effect of separating and breaking down blood clots.

Thrombophlebitis Inflammation of a vein accompanied by formation of a clot. It has a number of causes, including trauma to the wall of the vein, prolonged sitting, standing or immobilisation.

Thromboprophylaxis Measures taken to avoid the development of DVT, eg. the use of appropriate support hosiery and/or drugs, eg. heparin before and after surgery in 'at risk' groups.

Thrush (SEE Candida).

Tibial artery Distal branch of popliteal artery in the posterior knee.

Tincture Spirit/alcohol solution of a substance for painting on the skin's surface.

Tinea pedis Athlete's foot, a fungal infection frequently caused by dermatophytes or candida.

Tissue culture The maintenance and growth of pieces of explanted tissue in culture. Usually refers to the much more frequently used technique of cell culture, using cells dispersed from tissues.

Tissue engineering Construction of tissues outside the human body. In *in vitro* culture, it is impossible to achieve the three-dimensional structure found *in vivo*. A scaffold or dermal-like support must be produced to provide cells with an appropriate environment to grow to the required shape. Cultured dermis consists of neonatal dermal fibroblasts cultured *in vitro* on a biosorbable polyglactin (Vicryl) mesh. Used to replace damaged tissue with living, healthy dermal tissue consisting of collagen, fibronectin, glycosaminoglycans and growth factors.

Tissue tolerance The amount of pressure an individual can withstand before capillary occlusion. Tissue tolerance is reduced by many factors, eg. low blood pressure, malnutrition, sustained pressure, etc.

Tissue turgor Resilience and normal firmness expected on palpation of tissues.

Tissue viability The ability of tissue to perform its normal function optimally.

Tone Normal resilience and tension in, for example, skin or muscle.

Topical anaesthetic Anaesthetics such as lignocaine, amethocaine, or ethyl chloride may be applied topically in solution, gel or cream formulations to reduce pain. In Europe, cream anaesthetics are often used on chronic wounds but they are not licensed for this purpose in the UK.

Topical antibiotics Antibiotics incorporated into a dressing, powder or cream. There is a high potential for both patient and bacterial sensitivity and application of topical antibiotics is generally inadvisable.

Torsion Mechanical stress which has a rotation element.

Total contact plaster A frequent treatment for patients with diabetic foot ulceration. The wound is dressed and the lower limb encased in a plaster of Paris case to protect from trauma and provide even pressure distribution. Has the drawback of permanence, any developing infection will not be noticed until the plaster is removed. Recently, removable plastic equivalents have been introduced.

Toxins 'poisons'.

TNF (SEE Tumour necrosing factor).

Transcutaneous oxygen Oxygen levels in blood may be measured by an instrument applied to the skin (transcutaneous pO_2 monitor). This technique is often used to quantify ischaemia and hence tissue oxygen perfusion in patients with ulceration of the foot and lower limb. Low pO_2 is a measure of ischaemia in diabetic foot ulceration.

Transduction Transfer of genes by bacteriophages (virus). There is evidence that transduction can occur between species.

Transfoming growth factor (TGF) Transforming growth factors are proteins secreted by transformed cells that can stimulate the growth of normal cells. TGF alpha binds to the EGF receptor and exerts an angiogenic effect through the stimulation of microvascular endothelial cell growth. TGF beta stimulates wound healing.

Transpiration rate (SEE MVTR).

Trauma Wounds caused by injury, eg. lacerations, surgical incision and burns (or self-harm).

Traumatic wound (SEE Trauma).

Tri-phasic sound The normal three sounds heard on a handheld Doppler when assessing blood flow: the first is dilation of the blood vessel as a volume of blood passes through; the second is the recoil; and the third, rebound to normal vessel tone. (SEE Biphasic and monophasic.)

Trophic changes Occur when oxygen and nutrients are prevented from reaching the tissues.

Tulle Gras French term for an open weave fabric dressing impregnated with white soft paraffin. It has been widely used in the treatment of burns, donor sites and chronic wounds.

Tumour 1. May be a benign or malignant overgrowth of a tissue or organ. 2. Originally one of the four cardinal signs of inflammation — rubor, dolor, calor, and tumor; red, painful, hot, swollen. Some tumours may break through the skin 'fungate' and lead to a serious skin lesion.

Tumour necrosing factor A cytokine generated in any focus of inflammation. The main reason for cachexia in malignant tumours.

Turning clock A method of recording the times and frequency of patient repositioning.

Two-hourly turns Ritualistic practice for re-positioning patients in the prevention of pressure ulcers. Although it prevents pressure ulcers in a large number of immobile patients, there are many who require increased frequency of re-positioning, and two-hourly turns places these patients at high risk. There are also many patients who will experience pain when being moved or those who are dying and would wish peace. Repositioning times should be dictated by the individual patient's condition and the 30-degree tilt is a less traumatic method of repositioning. (SEE Thirty-degree tilt.)

U

Ulcer A lesion of the skin, which can be accompanied by necrotic tissue, and caused by a number of factors. A non-healing wound. (SEE Pressure ulcer and leg ulcer.)

Ultrasound imaging Ultrasonography. The use of high-frequency ultrasonic sound waves to examine interior structures of the body, such as the heart and vascular system, and for foetal monitoring.

Ultrasound Therapeutic ultrasound for treatment of soft tissue injury, sometimes used to treat chronic ulcers.

Unna's boot A method of compression used in the treatment of leg ulcers, particularly favoured in the USA. A rigid

boot is made by placing a layer of gelatin-glycerin-zinc oxide paste, and then applying a spiral bandage. Several more coats of paste are used to produce a boot. This impregnated bandage becomes rigid and provides a resistant case to the limb.

Ultraviolet light Part of the electro-magnetic spectrum beyond the violet range of visible light, may be used as a bacteriostatic.

Ungual Pertaining to the nail.

Urticaria Skin condition which appears like nettle stings, may be due to contact or drug allergy.

V

VAC (SEE Vacuum assisted closure).

Vacuum assisted closure (VAC)
The wound is fully occluded with adhesive film and suction is applied at 120 to 125mmHg. This can be continuous suction or intermittent. Bacteria and exudate are removed from the wound bed and stored in the suction holder. The resulting hypoxic environment is thought to encourage angiogenesis and negative pressure 'pulls' blood to the site. Critical colonisation will not occur in vacuum therapy as the bacteria are removed before reproduction can occur.

Validity A check to see if you are measuring what you want to measure, an important part of research rigour.

Vapour permeable Gases and water vapour can pass through, eg. a dressing surface.

Varicose eczema Skin condition associated with varicose veins characterised by itching, often skin scaling. Scratch lines (excoriation) may be visible.

Varicose ulcer Tissue breakdown occurs following build up of metabolites in the tissue and increased venous hypertension. This chronic ulcer often produces copious exudate and may have deep infection present, although superficial swabs show only the usual bacterial wound contaminants.

Varicose veins The valves in the leg veins become damaged due to either deep vein thrombosis or long periods of standing seen in certain occupations, such as hairdressing. The veins become engorged and are swollen. There may be a familial tendency to poor quality semilunar valves, which allow reflux of blood back down the vein, distending the distal lumen.

Varicosities (SEE Varicose veins).

Vascular An area of tissue consisting largely of blood vessels.

Vascular impairment Poor circulation of blood.

Vascular response May be dilation or contraction in response to a variety of stimuli, including temperature change, circulating blood volume changes, inflammatory state.

Vascularity The blood supply in an area of tissue.

Vasculitis Inflammation of blood vessels. Often found in patients with rheumatoid arthritis (*Figure 2*). Acutely painful. Treatment for vasculitis is steroid therapy. Wound dressings should be moist to 'bathe' nerve endings and reduce pain.

Vasoconstriction The arteries and arterioles constrict under the influence of drugs, hormones or cold.

Vasodilation The lumen of blood vessels opens and becomes wider, blood flow slows as a consequence, more oxygen can then dissociate into the tissues. Can cause flushing of the tissues.

Vasopressin A peptide hormone produced by the hypothalamus, which stimulates contraction of capillaries.

Venous Pertaining to the veins.

Venous hypertension When the veins become engorged (due to the inability of damaged valves to assist with blood return to the heart) the fluid creates a high pressure or tension within the lumen. When the calf muscle relaxes, the superficial venous system attempts to refill, but due to the increased pressure in the vein and the damaged valves, it is unable to do so fully. This leads to venous hypertension and a consequent potential for venous ulceration.

Venous insufficiency The valves in the superficial veins become inadequate due to possible deep vein thrombosis or long periods of standing. Because the valves no longer function effectively, plus the effect of gravity, blood collects in the lower limbs.

Venous obstruction oedema Deep vein thrombosis or tight stockings forming a tourniquet will prevent blood flow and increase potential for oedema distal to the obstruction.

Venous Occlusion Plethysmography (VOP) Venous occlusion, a specific and most common application of impedance plethysmography. Normally, a pressure cuff is used to close temporarily the veins. The rate at which the veins then fill or empty is measured in order to diagnose blood flow disturbances and occlusions. VOP can be used to diagnose deep vein thromboses, to evaluate post-thrombotic syndrome functionality, and to determine other functional parameters of the venous system.

Venous return The ability of the system to return blood to the heart. Blood return relies on the calf muscle pump and intra-thoracic pressure. On compression of tissues, the speed of the flow of blood from the capillary network back into the tissues was used in the past to provide an indication of capillary bed integrity, however, current advice is only to use this assessment information in conjunction with other assessment methods.

Venous stasis The blood pools in the lower extremities and becomes static when the patient is immobile (calf muscles are not 'pumping' the blood to the heart), or when the valves within the veins are ineffective and allow the blood to return to the lower extremities.

Virchow's triad In the 1860s Rudolf Virchow suggested that the factors that promote thrombus formation were in three categories, namely:

- ❖ changes in the composition of the blood
- ❖ changes in blood flow
- ❖ changes in the internal surface of the blood vessel.

We now know that the factors promoting thrombosis are complex involving platelet adhesion, release and aggregation. Virchow was not aware of the existence of the platelet but did, nevertheless, broadly cover the relevant factors.

Virulence Implies a microbe has marked pathological effects on the body.

Visco-elastic foam Cellular material which deforms under load, but restores on off-loading; may be used in insoles and seating to provide impact absorption. A key feature is that the foam responds and contours to the warmth of the body as well as deforming under load.

Vitamin C Vitamin C or ascorbic acid is essential for the formation of collagen and other tissue such as the skin, bone and connective tissue. Ascorbic acid aids healing in wounds. If a person is at risk of developing pressure ulcers, or has an established wound, a vitamin C supplement should be considered.

Vitiligo Skin condition characterised by patches of white skin (where no melanin is present) and darker skin.

Vitronectin Is a serum protein also called serum spreading factor because of its ability to promote adhesion and spreading of cells.

Voucher scheme Provided by NHS wheelchair services. The voucher scheme can be utilised by service users in order to purchase the wheelchair of their choice, within limitations.

W

Warfarin Anticoagulant (to inhibit clotting of blood). Prevents uptake of vitamin K (vital for clotting to occur) in the gut. Patients administered with warfarin will bleed easily (even haemorrhage) if the wound is disturbed by dry/inappropriate dressings or debridement.

Warmth Sense of comfortable heat, may be applied or perceived. Warmth is essential for wound healing. Any drop of temperature greater than 2°C can delay wound healing for up to four hours. A healing wound should have a dressing *in situ* for as long as possible to maintain the warmth. Cigarette smoking lowers the temperature of the skin and this may delay wound healing.

Wart Caused by the human papilloma virus. On the foot the bulk of extra hyper-plastic tissue is squashed into tissues by body weight, this lesion is also called a verruca (pl. verrucae), while on hands or legs, this benign tumour appears as a bump with a rough surface.

Water donating dressings Any dressing that contains water that is likely to increase fluid within the wound, eg. hydrogels.

Waterlow risk assessment A method of assessing risk of pressure ulcer development. Only meant as a tool to assist in assessment, not as replacement for clinical judgement (SEE *Appendix*). (SEE Risk assessment.)

Wet-to-dry Gauze is soaked in normal saline and then placed in the wound and allowed to dry. It is then removed. Necrotic tissue adheres to the gauze and then can be pulled free. This procedure can cause the patient considerable pain if analgesia is not adequate and there is an added danger of healthy tissue being pulled free at the same time. This treatment is no longer justified because of pain to patients, trauma to the wound and evidence supporting modern moist dressings.

Wheelchair A wheeled chair used for personal mobility. There are many types of wheelchair available, some of which are manual, ie. propelled by large wheels, and others which are powered, ie. propelled by battery.

Wheelchair service A service funded by the NHS, most Health Authorities have a wheelchair service, whose remit is to supply wheelchairs for those with long term mobility problems. Provision covers both wheelchairs and seating systems.

White-cell trapping theory A theory for the pathogenesis of leg ulcers. Capillary loops are blocked by trapped white blood cells which interferes with the circulation, producing ischaemia and aggravating trophic changes already occurring in the skin. The trapped white cells become activated, releasing inflammatory mediators, which alter capillary permeability and precipitate the leakage of fibrin and other large molecules.

Windsweeping A postural change characterised by both of the legs moving to one side of the chair, giving the appearance that they have been blown to one side. The outer leg contacts with the outer margins of the wheelchair, potentially placing the lateral aspect of the knee joint at risk from developing a pressure ulcer; the same leg also abducts and laterally rotates at the hip joint. The inner leg moves alongside the other, causing adduction and medial rotation at the hip joint, and placing the joint at risk of dislocation. The pelvis tends to rotate forwards on one side. The trunk faces in the same direction as the windsweeping, but compensates and re-aligns itself to face forwards.

Wound A break in the epidermis or dermis that can be related to trauma or to pathological changes within the skin or body.

Wound bed preparation An umbrella term for the clinical measures taken to remove the barriers to wound healing. This will involve amongst others the control of exudate, the removal of unhealthy tissue and the management of infection.

Wound contraction As the wound bed advances level with the healthy tissues, the epithelial cells will begin to migrate over the wound surface and require a mixture of fibrin and fibronectin in order to migrate freely at a rate of 0.5mm/day. Myofibroblasts contract and this draws the edges of the wound closer together.

Wound healing A dermal repair and regeneration process which occurs in several stages. The first phase of healing is the inflammatory phase when growth factors and macrophage activity is at its height. In a chronic wound, healing is halted and the wound requires stimulating into the inflammatory phase to initiate wound healing once more. This can be achieved through skilful and knowledgeable use of dressings and thorough wound bed preparation.

Wound maturation Tissue remodelling in the final stage of healing. Maturation involves wound contraction, full epithelialisation and reorganisation of the dermal connective tissues, which can continue for up to two years. Epithelial tissue will continue to migrate over the surface of raw and viable (moist) tissue within the wound — a reason for keeping the wound in a constant healing state with granulation rather than allowing bacterial contamination to promote slough and necrotic tissue. Even at this stage, macrophages are important to collagen lysis and synthesis and there will be a mass of fibrous tissue. Contractile fibroblasts (myofibroblasts) will pull the wound edges together and the wound will change its appearance to become pale or white (a scar). Tensile strength is increased, as the new immature collagen crosslinks and matures.

Wound repair (SEE Wound healing).

y

Yellow wound The stage of healing or non-healing is sometimes identified through wound colour. This is a subjective method and is not accurate but can be helpful in noting wound changes during assessment and documentation. A yellow wound (*Figure 31*) is generally a sloughy wound (*Figure 32*) and may require debridement before the healing process will commence (*Figure 30*). Slough is generally a mixture of fibrous tissue, necrotic tissue, dead white cells and dead bacteria. Because it is a 'slime', bacteria can hide within slough and proliferate successfully. (SEE Slough; also SEE Red wound, Black wound, Green wound, Pink wound.)

Z

Zinc (Zn) A mineral that is critical to healing and a component of many systems (such as the immune system) and a co-factor in collagen formation. The recommended nutritional intake for zinc is 7–9mg/day. Zinc compounds are incorporated into a variety of topical preparations that are thought to be of value to wound healing but are as yet unproven, eg. calomine, zinc oxide cream and paste.

Zinc paste bandage A plain weave cotton fabric bandage impregnated with zinc oxide for the treatment of leg ulcers. Zinc paste bandages are also combined with calomine, cold tar, and ichthammol. Patients should be patch tested prior to application of these products as they have a potential for hypersensitivity reaction. Recently, a sterile rayon stocking impregnated with zinc oxide ointment has become available for the compression treatment of chronic leg ulcers.

Useful addresses

Advances in Skin and Wound Care
www.woundcarenet.com/advances.htm

American Academy of Wound
Management
1255 23rd ST NW, Suite 200
Washington DC, 20037
USA
Tel: (202) 521 0368
Fax (202) 833 3636
e-mail: woundnet@aawm.org

British Journal of Nursing
Mark Allen Publishing Ltd
Croxted Mews
288 Croxted Road
London SE24 9BY
Tel: 020 8671 7521
www.internurse.com

European Tissue Repair Society
www.etrs.org

European Wound Management Association
PO Box 864
London SE1 8TT
e-mail: ewma@congress-consult.com

Institute of Wound Management
Johnson & Johnson
Coronation Road
Ascot
Berkshire SL5 9EY
Tel: 01344 871 100

PubMed
www.ncbi.nlm.hih.gov/PubMed/

Tissue Viability Society
Glanville Centre
Salisbury District Hospital
Salisbury
Wiltshire SP2 8BJ

Judy Waterlow
www.judywaterlow.fsnet.co.uk

World Wide Wounds
www.worldwidewounds.com

Wound Care Society
Box 170
Harford
Huntingdon
PE21 1PL
www.woundcaresociety.org/

Appendix

Braden risk assessment						
Score	Sensory	Moisture	Activity	Mobility	Nutrition	Friction and shear
1	Completely limited	Constantly moist	Bed-bound	Completely immobile	Very poor	Problem
2	Very limited	Very moist	Chair-bound	Very limited	Probably inadequate	Potential problem
3	Slightly limited	Occasionally moist	Walks occasionally	Slightly limited	Adequate	No apparent problem
4	No impairment	Rarely moist	Walks frequently	No limitations	Excellent	
A score of 16 or less indicates that a person is at risk of pressure ulcer development						

Norton risk assessment

Score	Physical condition	Mental condition	Activity	Mobility	Incontinence
4	Good	Alert	Ambulant	Full	Not
3	Fair	Apathetic	Walks with help	Slightly limited	Occasionally
2	Poor	Confused	Chair-bound	Very limited	Usually urine
1	Very bad	Stuporous	Bed-fast	Immobile	Doubly

A score of 14 or less indicates that a person is at risk of pressure ulcer development

Waterlow risk assessment

Body mass index	*	Skin type Visual risk areas	*	Sex Age	*	Special risks Tissue malnutrition	*
BMI 20–24 (average)	0	Healthy	0	Male	1	Terminal cachexia	
BMI 25–29.9 (medium)	1	Tissue paper	1	Female	2	Cardiac failure	
BMI 30–>40 (large)	2	Dry	1	14–49	1	Peripheral vascular	
BMI <20 (obese)	3	Oedematous	1	50–64	2	Disease	
Continence	*	Clammy (Temp ↑)	1	65–74	3	Anaemia	
		Discoloured	2	75–80	4	Smoking	
		Broken/spot	3	81+	5		
Complete/		**Mobility**	*	**Appetite**	*	**Neurological deficit**	*
catheterised	0					eg. Diabetes, MS,	
Occasion incont.	1	Fully	0	Average	0	CVA, motor/sensory,	
Cath/incontinent of		Restless/fidgety	1	Poor	1	paraplegia	5
faeces	2	Apathetic	2	NG tube/		Pain	
Doubly incont.	3	Restricted	3	fluids only	2	**Major surgery/**	*
		Inert/traction	4	NBM/		**trauma**	
		Chair-bound	5	anorexic	3		
						Orthopaedic —	
						below waist, spinal,	5
						on table >2 hours	5
Score						**Medication**	*
10+ At risk						Cytotoxics	
15+ High risk						High-dose steroids	
20+ Very high risk						Anti-inflammatory	4

Reproduced by kind permission of Judy Waterlow

Medley score pressure sore prevention
Risk assessment and protection chart

Patient details:

Name: _____   DOB: _____   Admission date: _____

Ward: _____   Diagnosis: _____

Risk assessment:

Assign a numerical value to each of the following categories:

	Assessments						
	date						
Activity — ambulation							
Ambulant without assistance	0						
Ambulant with assistance	2						
Chairfast (longer than 12 hours)	4						
Bedfast (longer than 12 hours)	6						
Mobility — range of movement							
Full active range of movement	0						
Moves with limited assistance	2						
Moves only with assistance	4						
Immobile	6						
Skin condition							
Healthy	0						
Rashes or abrasions	2						
Advanced age (65+) dehydrated	4						
Oedema and/or redness	6						
Pressure sore involved	6						
Grade of sore (see below)							
Predisposing diseases							
None	0						
Chronic stable	1						
Acute or chronic stable	2						
Terminal	3						

Risk assessment:	Assessments						
Level of consciousness	date						
Alert	0						
Lethargic/confusion	1						
Semi-comatosed (responds to stimuli)	2						
Comatosed (absence of response to stimuli)	3						
Nutritional status							
Good (TPN or naso gastric feeds)	0						
Fair (insufficient intake to maintain weight)	1						
Poor (eats/drinks very little)	2						
Very poor (unable or refuses to eat; emaciated)	3						
Incontinence — bladder							
Total control/catheterised	0						
Occasional (less than 2 x per 24 hours)	1						
Usually (more than 2 x per 24 hours)	2						
Total control	3						
Incontinence — bowel							
Total control	0						
Occasional (less than 2 x per 24 hours)	1						
Usually (more than 2 x per 24 hours)	2						
Total (no control)	3						
Pain (patient's report)							
None	0						
Mild	1						
Intermittent	2						
Severe	3						
	Total						
Initials							

Patient risk score		Patient support selection
0–9	Low risk	Protect heels
10–19	Medium risk	Pressure relieving mattress
20–36	High risk	Dynamic flotation up to air fluidised therapy

Grade 1 — skin is likely to break down. Red/black blister
Grade 2 — superficial break in the skin
Grade 3 — destruction of skin without cavity
Grade 4 — destruction of skin with cavity